THE
POSTNATAL
EXERCISE
BOOK

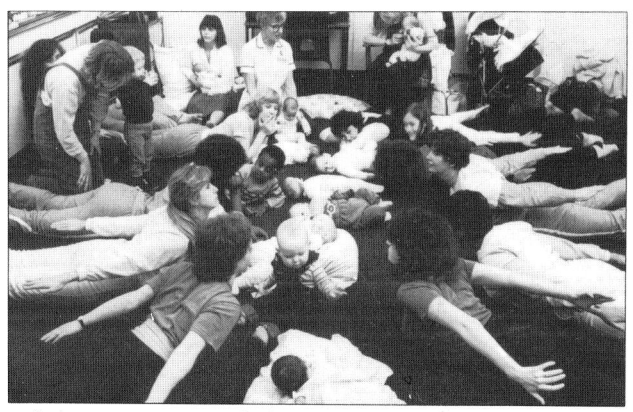

*A program of fitness and well-being
for mother and baby*

THE
POSTNATAL
EXERCISE
BOOK

A program of fitness and well-being for mother and baby

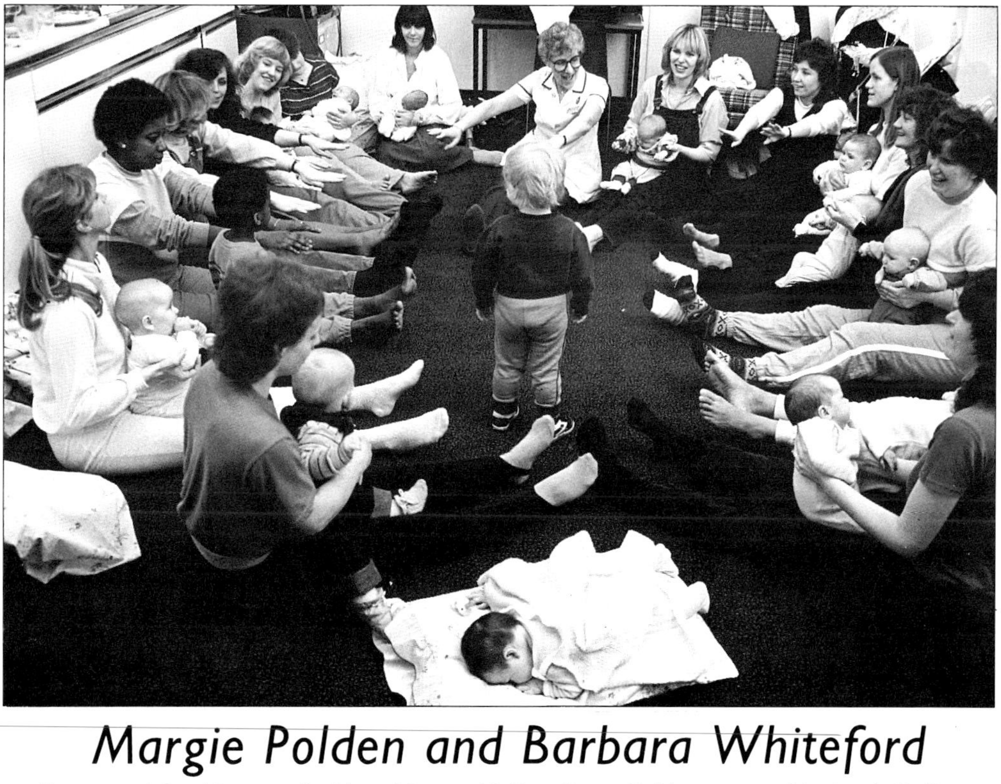

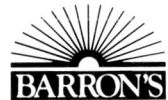

Margie Polden and Barbara Whiteford

Foreword by Harvey S. Marchbein, M.D., Cornell University Medical College

Photographs by Sandra Lousada

BARRON'S

Published in the United States in 1992 by Barron's Educational Series, Inc.

Copyright © 1992, 1984 by Frances Lincoln Limited,
Apollo Works, 5 Charlton Kings Road, London, England.
Text copyright © 1992, 1984 by Margie Polden and Barbara Whiteford.
Photographs copyright © 1992, 1984 by Sandra Lousada.
Illustrations copyright © 1992, 1984 by Frances Lincoln Limited.

All inquiries should be addressed to:
Barron's Educational Series, Inc.
250 Wireless Boulevard
Hauppauge, New York 11788

First published in Great Britain by Century Hutchinson Limited 1984.
Reprinted 1987, 1985; revised edition 1988, reprinted 1990.
First Frances Lincoln (second revised) edition September 1992.

Library of Congress Catalog Card No. 91-42911
International Standard Book No. 0-8120-4993-4

Library of Congress Cataloging-in-Publication Data
Polden, Margie
   The postnatal exercise book: a program of fitness and well-being for new
mothers / Margie Polden & Barbara Whiteford; foreword by Harvey S.
Marchbein, M.D.; photographs by Sandra Lousada.
   p.   cm.
   Includes bibliographical references and index.
   ISBN 0-8120-4993-4
   1. Postnatal care. 2. Exercise for women 3. Physical fitness
for women.
I. Whiteford, Barbara. II. Title.
RG801.W7   1992
613.7'045—dc20   91-42911
                                                  CIP

PRINTED IN HONG KONG

CONTENTS

FOREWORD

Our perceptions of pregnancy and our attitude toward pregnant and postnatal women have shifted remarkably during the past few years. Not long ago, women's activities were severely restricted during pregnancy and they were instructed to avoid undue physical stress under all circumstances. When it came time to give birth, instead of enjoying the emotional benefit of having a baby at home, women delivered their children in the more sterile environment of the hospital. There, the physical risk of delivery was reduced but the emotional support parents could give each other was drained from the experience. Mothers and fathers were separated for an extended period of time. After the baby arrived following a normal vaginal delivery, mothers spent a week resting in the hospital. Once they got home, it was standard practice to keep new mothers in bed and severely restrict their physical activity.

All this is changing. Our perspective has undergone revolutionary alterations. Pregnancy is no longer considered a disease requiring inordinate bed rest. Our patients are kept active and they work at looking and feeling their vibrant best. Research has shown that this new practice is not only safe but conveys many benefits. This new active attitude has both mental and physical advantages for women throughout their pregnancy, labor, delivery and postnatal experiences.

That's why, nowadays, our patients stay in the hospital for only a few short days after delivery—frequently for less than forty-eight hours. They return home to run their households, care for their children, and, in many instances, return to work outside the home fairly quickly. Even after delivering by Caesarean, women are impatient to resume their crucial role in family life. Consequently, women who undergo Caesarean sections are also on their feet sooner and what used to be a post-operative hospital stay of seven or eight days, now has been shortened to three or four.

All of these changes are signs of a new and innovative attitude toward postnatal recuperation. After giving birth, women are anxious to regain control of their bodies as soon as possible. In a society where so many women now do work outside and/or within the home, it is imperative that they do so. To accomplish this, they also need to know how to be as physically comfortable as possible.

At the same time as our attitude toward pregnancy has

evolved, our scientific knowledge about the relationship between weight control and exercise has also expanded, fueled by an intense public interest in the subject. And for a public obsessed with physical fitness and health, the up-to-date information on postnatal care found in *The Postnatal Exercise Book* plays a vital role.

The Postnatal Exercise Book not only describes a wide range of useful exercises, it also describes the emotional and physical changes women can expect during this period. It includes activities for both the new mother and her newborn. And the book contains invaluable advice for a population of new mothers that increasingly includes women of vastly different ages and physical conditions.

Until recently, the only exercises given to postnatal women were for strengthening and toning the vaginal muscles—as though these were the only muscles affected by giving birth. A more general approach is called for. A woman's entire body undergoes significant changes while carrying a fetus for nine months and all of the body's muscles have to adjust to the change in posture as the abdomen grows in size. Even after delivery, it is not enough to assume that time alone will take care of your body. A good mental attitude and a safe exercise program will enhance your body's efficient recovery from the rigors of pregnancy and delivery.

Obstetricians know that our patients are enthusiastically ready to do what is necessary to regain control of their bodies and their lives. Many patients now take prenatal exercise classes to stay in good physical shape during pregnancy. There's no reason for them to stop exercising after they give birth.

When society changes its mind about something, we're frequently told to "get with the program!" It's high time that we got with the program in the way we treat postnatal women— encouraging them to embrace an active and healthy lifestyle. Thanks to *The Postnatal Exercise Book*, that program is now available to every woman. Enjoy it and your newborn in good health.

Harvey S. Marchbein, M.D.
Department of Obstetrics and Gynecology,
North Shore University Hospital –
Cornell University Medical College

INTRODUCTION

The drama of birth is the climax of long months of waiting and preparation for all women. Lying there with your new baby, you may feel energetic, relieved, and euphoric, or perhaps exhausted, anxious, and sore. You might have been prepared for the wide-ranging and varying intensity of moods that are an inevitable part of becoming a mother, but possibly you thought that your body at least would return to normal very soon after your baby was born. You watched with pride your blooming, expanding abdomen and breasts as pregnancy advanced, but now the birth is over, you expect to find yourself back as you were. Instead you are faced with another body; a flabby, bulging abdomen with crêpey skin and maybe some stretch marks, a weak pelvic floor; a weary, drooping body you barely recognize.

Although you may only just be beginning to learn how much has to be done for your small, utterly dependent baby, you also begin to realize that you will need to do something positive for yourself to return to the way you were. For nine months your body was adapting to a growing baby; fortunately, it should not take nearly so long to restore it. Some of the changes occur within hours of your baby's birth: the uterus starts contracting down immediately, returning to normal by about six weeks; you also lose a large amount of tissue fluid in the days immediately following delivery. Even so, your muscles need time and help to return to their normal strength and function, and how quickly this happens depends largely on you.

Using the exercises

The exercises in this book are carefully graded to be useful from immediately after the birth to six months later, and are designed to strengthen those muscles that have suffered most as a result of pregnancy and labor. Even though your ligaments are still softened by the pregnancy hormones, gently exercising and strengthening muscles compensates and helps protect your body against the demands of caring for your new baby.

Avoiding long-term problems starts now: strong abdominal muscles protect the back; strong thigh muscles support the knee;

and strong pelvic floor muscles (also called "Kegel exercises") help prevent future stress from incontinence and prolapse. (Exercising the pelvic floor muscles can be regularly done anywhere, anytime, and is essential.)

These exercises are suitable for most women regardless of age, shape, current fitness, and type of labor. However, before beginning any exercise program, it is important to check with your doctor, especially if you have a history of any back or joint problems.

Arranging your exercise schedule

The three sections (0–6 weeks, 6 weeks to 3 months, 3–6 months) offer a rough guide, designed for the average woman. If you exercised regularly right up to delivery, then you can progress to the second and third stages earlier than suggested. If you had a Caesarean section, or took very little exercise before and during pregnancy, you will need to spend longer on the early exercises before moving onto the next stage. Useful ways of assessing your progress are to test the strength of your important muscles (see pages 52 and 99). Remember, too, that even if you didn't begin any exercises immediately, it is never too late to start.

If this is your first baby you may be surprised just how totally absorbing, and possibly frustrating, you find your new role. You cannot hear a baby's cry without assuming that it must be yours; you cannot go out for more than a few minutes for fear that you will be needed, and you strongly believe that no one else can comfort your baby. All these feelings are normal and natural and probably ensure that mothers satisfy their babies' many needs. Any program of exercises must not, therefore, force you into unwanted and uncomfortable separation from your baby, so most of the exercises in this book are designed to be done at home.

Helping your baby's development

Alongside your own exercises, there are recommended positions, handling, and play for your baby at the relevant stages of development. Just as in labor, when knowledge enabled you to direct your energy to coping with it, if you are informed and confident in handling your baby, you will be more relaxed and fulfilled as a mother, and your baby will feel more secure and contented in your care.

Rest and relaxation

Rest and relaxation are as vital as exercise so it is important at the start of your program to be sensible and flexible about it. If you have been up all night and feel exhausted, then postpone your exercise session until you have had a rest. If you feel energetic, repeat the appropriate exercises, taking care not to overdo it as you will do more harm than good. Observe your body's response and remember, exercise should feel comfortable and make you feel good. Bear in mind too that you have just been through one of the most physically exhausting and strenuous events of your life and that your body needs time to recuperate.

YOUR BODY
BEFORE AND AFTER
THE BIRTH

During pregnancy, you have undergone gradual changes to your body, posture, and emotions, yet within the few hours of labor you will have given birth to your baby and will have begun to experience a whole new range of changes. Some begin restoring your body to its former state, and others help you provide the necessary love, food, and care for your baby.

These postnatal changes are quite dramatic: naturally it does not take as long for the body to return to its pre-pregnancy state as it does to nurture a developing fetus from a single cell to an eight pound baby. In order to understand how your body recovers and to see where exercise can help, it is useful to familiarize yourself with your anatomy and to look at the way it is affected by both pregnancy and birth.

The pelvic girdle

The pelvic girdle is made up of four sets of bones; the first and most obvious are the big hip bones, which join in front at the symphysis pubis. They curve upward to form two bony wings (the ilia) just beneath your waist, and downward to give you the bones you sit on. Wedged between these at the back is the sacrum (the base of the spine), joined to the hip bones at the sacroiliac joints. Finally, there is the coccyx, the remains of the human tail.

Like all the other joints of the body, the pelvic joints are held together by ligaments. Normally little or no movement takes place in them, but during pregnancy special hormones gradually soften your body's ligaments, so that they stretch slightly. This enables both the entrance and exit of the pelvis to increase in size as your baby passes through during labor. It will take five to six months for your ligaments to recover normal firmness.

Curving between the sacrum and the head are the twenty-four bones of the spine. If you put one hand on your symphysis pubis, and the other on your sacrum, you will feel that the distance from back to front is not very great; in fact, the internal diameter of the pelvis from back to front is only 4–5 in (10–12 cm).

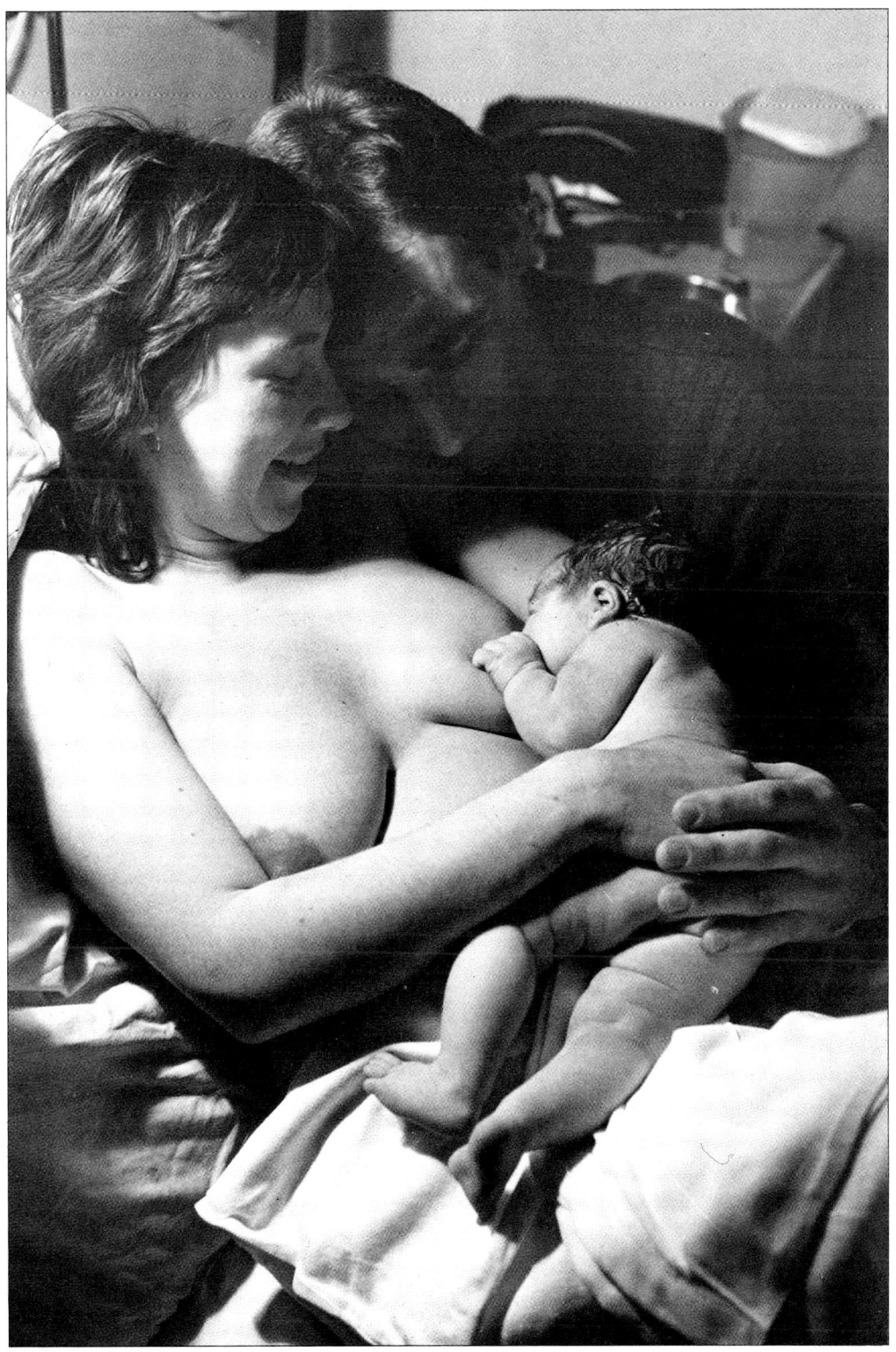

The pelvic girdle

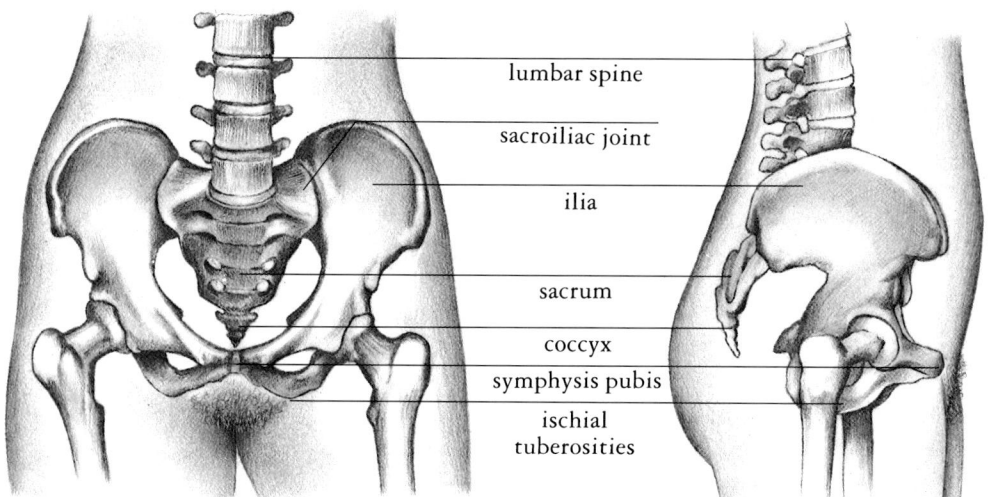

lumbar spine

sacroiliac joint

ilia

sacrum

coccyx

symphysis pubis

ischial tuberosities

Usually your pelvic organs – bladder, uterus, and rectum – fit comfortably into this space, but by the end of your pregnancy the baby in the uterus makes things a tight squeeze.

The ligaments

Ligaments are inelastic bands of supportive tissue that help hold your joints together. During pregnancy the ligaments soften and stretch due to the influence of the hormones progesterone and relaxin, resulting in some increase in movement in all your joints, not just your pelvic girdle. The effects of these changes can persist for some time after your baby is born, and may be felt as aching or sometimes pain, especially in the joints of your back and the joints between your spine and pelvis (your sacroiliac joints). Occasionally this will radiate into your buttock or leg. The joint in the front of your pelvis (the symphysis pubis) can give rise to problems as well.

The uterus

The uterus is a muscular bag that normally weighs about 2–3 oz (50–70 g), and fits snugly into your pelvic girdle along with the other organs. By the end of your pregnancy the uterus alone weighs about 2.2 lb (1 kg).

Involution

Immediately after the birth your uterus can be felt through your soft abdominal wall just below the umbilicus. It is about the size it was at the fifth month of pregnancy. It starts to contract down straight away – the process known as involution – returning to its former size and position by six weeks. These contractions may initially be felt as "after pains," which will be more pronounced if you already have one or more children. At first, breastfeeding stimulates these contractions, which can feel like period pains or the discomfort felt in very early labor. The deep, relaxing breathing exercise on page 49 will help you cope with this uncomfortable but natural process of recovery.

The blood forced out by your contracting uterus from the raw

The pelvic organs

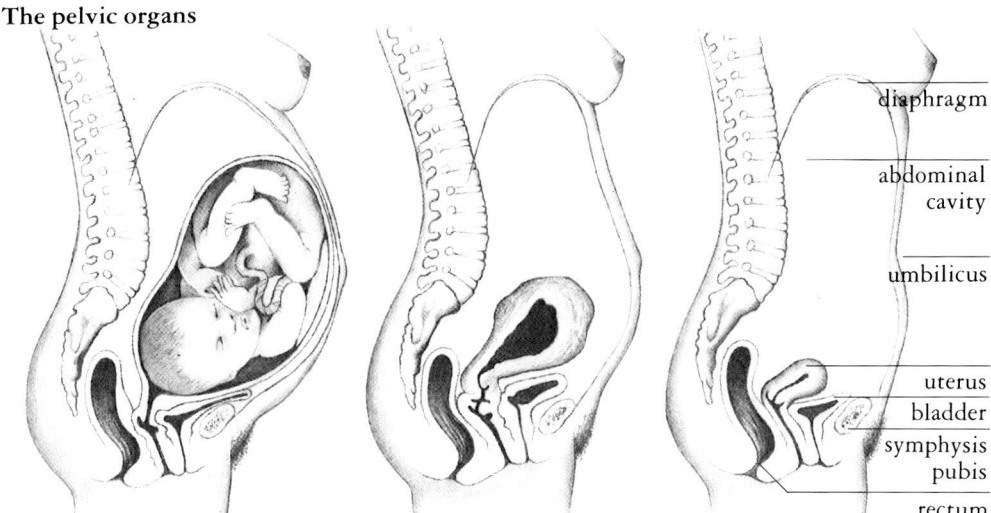

diaphragm

abdominal cavity

umbilicus

uterus
bladder
symphysis pubis
rectum

At the end of pregnancy
Because of your bulging abdomen, your posture alters and the organs are compressed

Immediately after the birth
You will probably still look about six months pregnant.

Six weeks after the birth
Your uterus should have contracted down to its normal shape, size, and position.

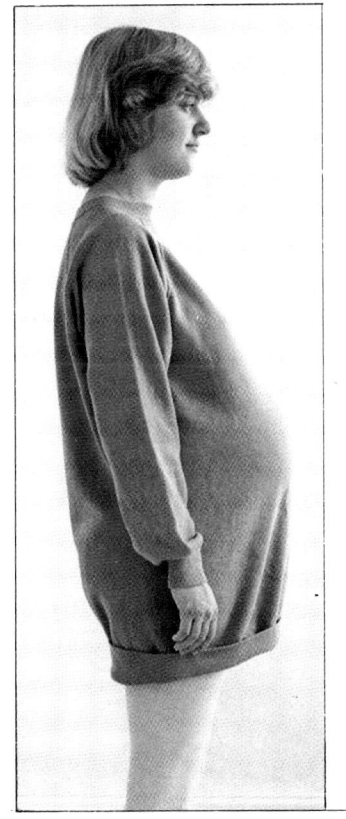
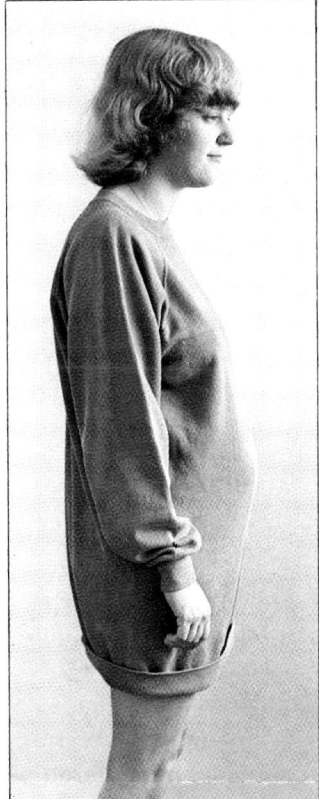
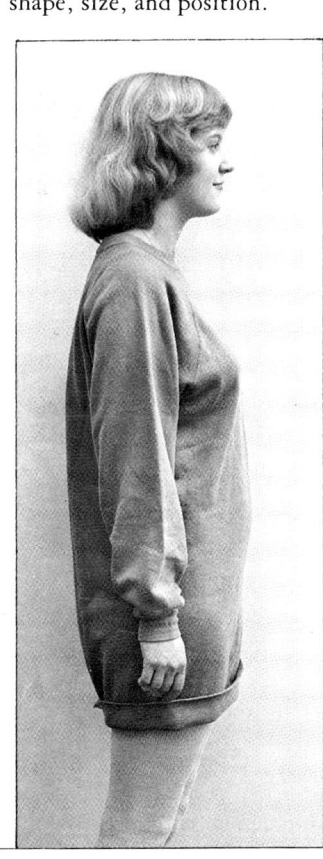

site of the placenta is called the lochia. It should be red for the first few days, gradually changing to brown, then yellow, and finally disappearing between two to six weeks. You should report any large clots, sudden heavy loss, or offensive smell to your doctor.

Within a week or so of the birth it should no longer be possible to feel your uterus in your abdomen, as it has shrunk down into your pelvis (though it is still larger than normal). When you go for your postnatal examination, your doctor will check to make sure your uterus has fully contracted.

The pelvic floor

Helping to support your pelvic organs is a hammock of muscle known as the pelvic floor, which is enormously stretched by childbirth. The pelvic floor muscles are divided into a deep and a superficial layer and have three openings: the urethra (from the bladder); the vagina (from the uterus); and the anus (from the bowel). The muscle fibers surround each of these openings in a figure eight, the front part looping around the vagina and urethra and the back part around the anus; however, they work as one complete unit. Some of the muscle fibers are able to work

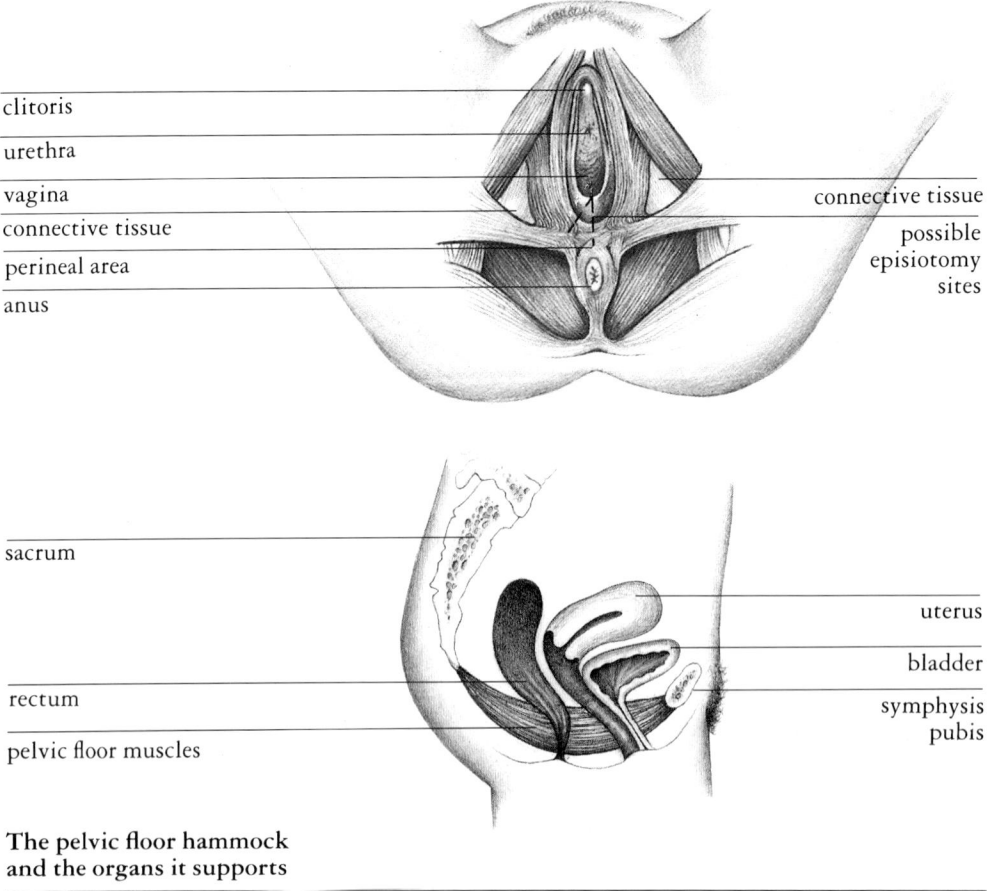

clitoris

urethra

vagina

connective tissue

perineal area

anus

connective tissue

possible episiotomy sites

sacrum

uterus

bladder

rectum

symphysis pubis

pelvic floor muscles

The pelvic floor hammock and the organs it supports

strongly over long periods, while others can only work in short bursts, as when you cough or sneeze. The wedge of muscles between the vagina and the anus is known as the perineum. If you have an episiotomy to assist the safe delivery of your baby, this is where it will be. Tears can also occur here and in the vagina.

The muscles making up the pelvic floor are held together by sheets of non-stretchy tissue called fascia. Before pregnancy, most women are completely unaware of these muscles, yet they are very important for health and comfort because they support the pelvic organs and prevent the bladder and bowel from leaking. Strong pelvic floor muscles can also improve the quality of your sex life.

During pregnancy, the pelvic floor will have had to carry the increased weight of your baby and uterus; during the second stage of labor, it will have thinned out and stretched open around your baby's head and body. This stretching can numb or damage the nerve fibers that supply the pelvic floor muscles so that, initially, there may be a loss of sensation and you will not be able to feel your muscles contract. This usually improves gradually but long-term damage can occur to your nerves, and therefore to your muscles, too. It is most important to make sure that you properly regain the full use of your pelvic floor muscles. If you can't feel them working, look in a small mirror or, later, feel with two fingers in your vagina, to reassure yourself. After six weeks, if you are still not able to contract your pelvic floor muscles, consult your doctor for full assessment and advice. The pelvic floor may also have been damaged by an episiotomy or a tear, and many women experience pain, swelling, and bruising in this area for several days and are afraid to use their pelvic floor muscles.

If you have had stitches following a large tear or episiotomy, you may need to take mild painkillers for a while. The wound should be kept as clean and dry as possible by frequent bathing and changing of sanitary napkins. Your doctor may recommend hot sitz baths to relieve the pain and may also show you how to use ice to reduce swelling and relieve pain. A handful of crushed ice or some frozen peas in a polyethylene bag, wrapped in a clean, damp disposable gauze swab can be used when you are at home. Hold the ice pack against your perineum for five to ten minutes, three to four times a day.

Frequent pelvic floor "squeezes" are the best self-help method of relieving pain and promoting healing. Five contractions every five to ten minutes will soon ease the swelling and feeling of stiffness. After a few days, the swelling and discomfort should have subsided.

If you have had an episiotomy or tear it may help you overcome any anxieties you have if you look at it in a mirror after a few days. You will probably be surprised how well bonded the wound looks.

Three common
problems

1 **Sitting down** Sometimes perineal pain is so severe that women try to feed their babies standing up! Sitting well back on your chair or on two folded pillows with a gap between them can prove helpful. Make sure you put the part of you that is sorest in the gap between the pillows.

2 **Coughing, sneezing, or laughing** As you cough, a lot of pressure is exerted on your pelvic floor and it can feel as if your stitches are bursting. It is much more comfortable if you remember to squeeze in and lift your pelvic floor muscles when you cough, sneeze, blow your nose, or laugh (see page 52). Supporting your stitches with your hand over your pad can help too.

3 **Bowel movements** You will *not* tear your stitches if you have to strain to move your bowels. Holding a soft pad of clean toilet paper against them as you bear down will relieve pain.

If discomfort and pain persist when you walk, sit, stand, or, later, make love, be sure to mention it to your doctor when you have your postnatal checkup. If external scar tissue is causing problems, therapeutic ultrasound, administered by a physiotherapist, may soften it.

Bladder problems

Childbirth often affects the bladder; the following problems may occur.

Stress incontinence

Stress incontinence is uncontrollable leakage of small amounts of urine from your bladder when you cough, laugh, sneeze, or blow your nose, when you pick up something heavy, or perhaps run for a bus. It may have troubled you during your pregnancy; it may be something that developed after your baby was born. Pelvic tucks (see page 52) can help resolve this problem. Practice this inward and upward squeeze regularly: once or twice a day is *not* enough. Aim to have several pelvic floor exercise sessions a day. A good idea is to practice while feeding your baby. Initially you may have very poor sensation around the vagina but it should gradually return to normal and you should be able to feel these muscles working together, lifting inward and upward. Use the pelvic floor "squeeze" while coughing or blowing your nose to try and control the leakage. As you breathe in to cough, quickly draw the pelvic floor in and up; hold it tightly braced until the cough is over, and only then relax.

Although stress incontinence can often be cured by correct and conscientious exercising, it is most important to know if you are doing the pelvic floor exercise correctly. If you are not sure, ask your doctor to refer you to a specialist who will assess the strength of your muscles and can also offer a variety of other treatments. If these are unsuccessful, your doctor may suggest a repair operation if your internal ligaments and supporting tissues have been badly stretched.

Urgency

During the first few days your body will rid itself of the extra fluid produced during pregnancy, and you will need to pass large amounts of urine fairly frequently. Many new mothers find it difficult to control the sudden urge to empty their bladder and sometimes accidents occur before reaching the bathroom. This is caused by a combination of bruising to the bladder and urethra during labor, and extreme weakness and "numbness" in the pelvic floor. Until your muscles are strong enough to give a really strong "squeeze" (this will calm down the feeling of urgency), when your bladder feels about to burst, press your hand against your perineum to help control your bladder.

Retention of urine   Sometimes it is difficult or impossible to empty the bladder after a baby is born. Useful strategies to help your bladder function normally are: pouring warm water over your perineum while you sit on the toilet, running a tap, or passing urine in the bathtub. If none of these efforts work, you will need a catheter to empty your bladder for a short time.

Bowel problems   Bowel problems sometimes occur after the birth, and although uncomfortable, or a nuisance, can often be alleviated.

Fecal incontinence   Very occasionally childbirth damages the nerves and muscles that control your anus so that you are unable to retain gas, and, sometimes, feces. Once again, correct pelvic floor exercising helps to correct this problem.

Constipation   During pregnancy, the hormones that soften your ligaments also relax the smooth muscles of your intestines so that they are not as efficient as they used to be at expelling their contents. Also, some iron pills are constipating and once your baby is born, an additional factor comes into play – your loose and floppy abdominal muscles give very poor support to the intestines and bowel. If you have had stitches and are taking painkillers, these, too, may cause constipation.

Another cause of postnatal constipation is simply fear of straining or tearing stitches in the perineum. Gently supporting your stitches with a pad of toilet paper as you bear down to move your bowels should make you more confident.

If you are constipated it is very important to eat fiber-rich foods, such as wholegrain bread, bran cereals, fresh fruit (do not peel apples and pears), celery, cabbage, and so on. You can add bran to your soups, stewed fruit, or yogurt – and be sure to drink extra fluid too. If, in spite of a sensible diet, you are still troubled by constipation, ask your doctor to recommend safe medication.

Hemorrhoids   Hemorrhoids, or piles, are swollen varicose veins in your rectum and anus. Sometimes they appear in pregnancy, sometimes after the baby is born – pushing in the second stage of labor can make them worse. They can be very painful, making sitting down very difficult. Your pelvic floor exercising will help by improving the circulation in this sensitive area and therefore reducing the pain. A crushed ice pack gently applied to the grapelike swelling can also give relief, and there are anesthetic ointments that your doctor can prescribe. Resting on your front (see page 53) and feeding your baby lying on your side will help. Hemorrhoids usually resolve after a short while.

Sexual problems

There is no "normal" time to resume sexual intercourse. Some women prefer to wait until the lochia is finished, but you may feel desire as early as seven days or not until seven months after your baby's birth, or even longer.

When you do both feel like trying intercourse, you may find it is very painful. Using a lubricating gel could help your partner achieve a gentler penetration, and trying another position might make a difference to the discomfort in your vagina and breasts. If you both lie on your sides or you lie or sit above your partner, then you will be able to control his penetration and the pressure on your tender breasts and perineum.

Sex is not just a matter of physical comfort, of course, and you may find that your feelings about it seem to change after the birth (see page 35). Guilt about this apparent change, fear of pain or damage to the perineum, anxiety about becoming pregnant again, or simply tiredness and preoccupation with your baby can all affect your desire for sex. You may also feel flabby, overweight, and unattractive. It is far better to try to talk these things through with your partner rather than keeping your feelings repressed. After all, there are many other ways of showing love apart from sexual intercourse.

If you are concerned that intercourse has been or will be painful or impossible, when you go for your postnatal checkup at about six weeks, do not be afraid to mention it to your doctor. Your perineum and vagina should be checked for healing, the strength of your pelvic floor muscles assessed, and your cervix examined to exclude the presence of a cervical erosion (ulcer) that could be a cause of pain during lovemaking. If your vaginal opening is found to be too tight, it can be treated – perhaps by gentle stretching. If you find that, far from a vagina that is too tight, it now feels loose and floppy so that neither of you gets any pleasure from intercourse, you should mention this too. It may be that an intensive regime of pelvic floor exercises will cure this, but if not, then a minor surgical repair may be recommended to correct the problem.

It is perfectly possible to become pregnant again very soon after giving birth, especially if you do not breastfeed. Decide which method of contraception you want to use *before* making love so that you are prepared. Discuss it with your doctor either in the hospital or at your postnatal checkup.

The abdominal muscles

One of the first things a mother does after her delivery is to feel her abdomen and notice how flat it seems and yet how flabby. This is because the abdominal muscles that have been stretched around the uterus do not of course immediately return to their original shape – and will not do so properly without help.

The muscle layers

Your abdominal "corset" consists of four layers of muscles. There are two superficial muscles – the recti abdominis – running straight up and down in front; two pairs of oblique muscles; and one pair of transverse muscles on each side. The muscles join down the midline, where a strip of fibrous tissue

Changes in the abdominal muscles

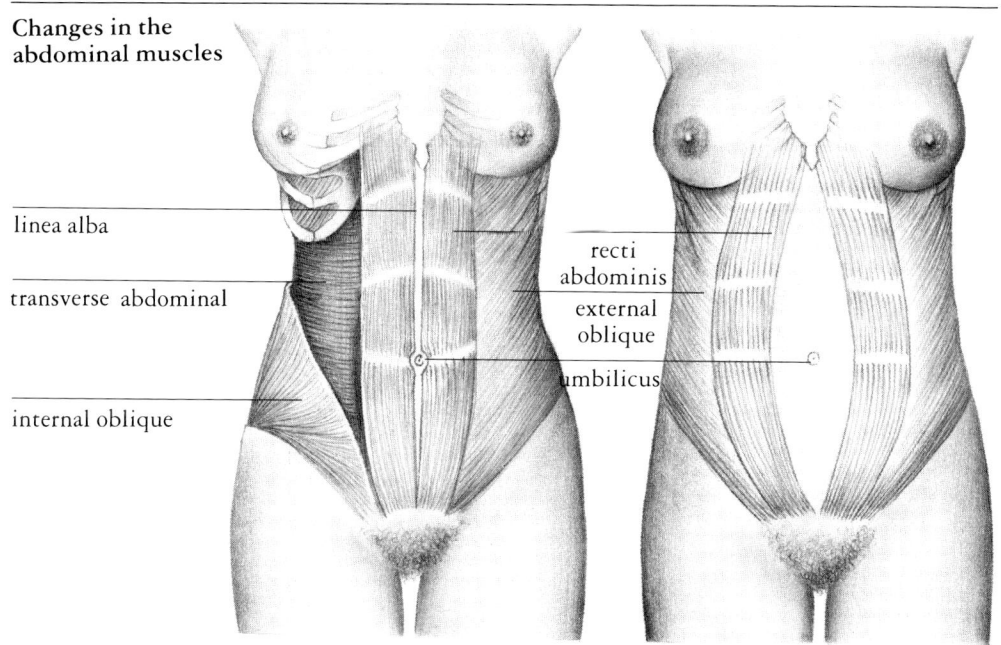

linea alba

transverse abdominal

internal oblique

recti abdominis

external oblique

umbilicus

Before pregnancy   After the birth

called the linea alba – normally about ½ in (1 cm) wide – can actually be seen on thin, muscular women before pregnancy. The abdominal muscles are weakest in the front, where they are only one layer deep.

How the muscles stretch

During pregnancy the abdominal muscles stretch and lengthen around the growing uterus; a woman who normally measures about 13 in (33 cm) from breastbone to pubis can stretch to around 20 in (50 cm), while her waist might increase from 26 in (66 cm) to 46 in (101 cm)! As the body's ligaments soften during pregnancy, the linea alba also softens; in late pregnancy it is quite common for the two recti to separate above and below the umbilicus. Unless they are very thin, few women realize this is happening because this condition – known as diastasis recti abdominis – is completely painless. Prolonged pushing in the second stage of labor in an uncomfortable position can increase this "gapping." Stretched and weak abdominal muscles will not be able to support your back properly, which could cause or increase backache.

Multiple births

If you had more than one baby, your abdominal muscles will be weaker and the separation between the recti will be greater, so that it will probably take much longer to reach full recovery. A new mother with one baby often finds that six to eight weeks pass before she has time to devote regularly to strengthening weak muscles; mothers of two or even more new babies will invariably be too tired and busy to exercise until perhaps three or more months have passed. No matter how long it is before you are able to start, you should be aware that it is *never too late*.

Structure of the breasts

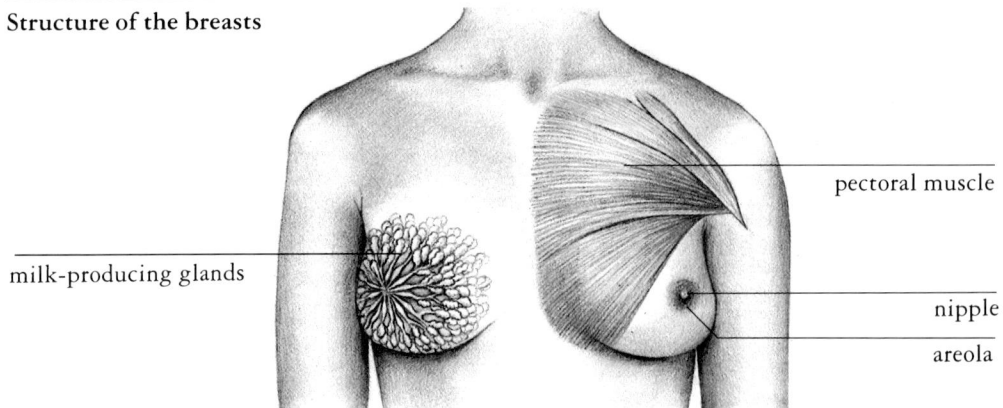

pectoral muscle

milk-producing glands

nipple

areola

The breasts

The major change in breast size occurs in pregnancy. The breasts are neither muscle nor ligament; they are mainly fat with a small amount of glandular tissue. Your breasts will have enlarged so that your bra size may have increased substantially. By the end of your pregnancy some of the fat under the skin of the breasts will have been absorbed, the milk-producing glands will have grown and developed, and you may have noticed the first few drops of colostrum, the substance that precedes true breast milk.

Production of milk

After your baby is delivered, the changing hormones stimulate your breasts to produce milk. True milk, the ideal food that also helps protect your baby from infection, does not "come in" until around the third day and until then the breasts continue to produce protein-rich colostrum. As the breasts begin to produce milk they become firm, large, and heavy, and as your baby feeds or you express the milk, a further supply is stimulated. Within a few weeks the supply and your baby's demands will probably coincide and your breasts will be softer.

If you are breastfeeding you may feel more comfortable if you wear a well-supporting bra. However, although there are no exercises for the breasts themselves it is certainly possible to improve the strength of the pectorals (their supporting muscles) and your posture, which is probably the most important factor in determining the position of your breasts on the chest wall. If you stand, sit, or walk with rounded shoulders your breasts are more likely to droop. Keep your back straight, lift your ribs, and remember to keep your shoulders down and relaxed. This will keep your breasts higher. Using the pectoral muscles vigorously will improve circulation and so may help lactation. Breastfeeding is a process that needs to be learned by mother and baby over a period of time. Common problems, such as sore nipples, can often be prevented or cured by positioning your baby correctly. Consult your doctor if you are having any problems.

The back, buttocks, and legs

After the birth, it is extremely important to have strong back, buttock, leg, and arm muscles, as any weakness may lead to poor posture, bad lifting techniques, and eventual backache. This is so important that a whole chapter has been devoted to it (see page 22).

Your legs may have become heavier in pregnancy, especially if you suffered from edema (fluid retention). Using and exercising your leg muscles will improve the circulation and lessen the swelling.

The average weight gain in pregnancy is about 28 lb (12.5 kg), although some women put on less and others much more. At least 10 lb (4.5 kg) of this will be fat on the hips, thighs, arms, back, and abdomen.

Weight loss

After delivery you will have lost the weight of your baby, the amniotic fluid, and the placenta – probably about 7–11 lb (3–5 kg). You may lose an extra 2–3 lb (1–1.5 kg) over the next few days as you excrete excess fluid from both tissues and extra blood volume. The uterus gradually shrinks from 2.2 lb (1 kg) to about 2–3 oz (50–70 g) during the next six weeks. However, you will probably find you are still heavier than you were before you became pregnant – maybe considerably so. This difference in weight is made up of fat.

Diet

If you are breastfeeding, some of this fat may be broken down to help produce breast milk and you may also be burning much of it up simply by doing the endless jobs involved in being a mother. However, just as it was during pregnancy, it is a myth that if you are breastfeeding you must eat for two. Your body seems to become more efficient and conserves energy during pregnancy and breastfeeding, so it is really the quality and not the quantity of food that will help to provide an adequate amount of milk. Avoid the "empty calories" contained in sweets such as ice cream, candy, cakes, and cookies. A well-balanced diet should include protein foods, such as eggs, meat and fish or beans, and other legumes, dairy foods, fruit, vegetables, fiber, and limited carbohydrate. Try and reduce the amount of fat in your diet – butter, margarine, cheese, cream, fat meat, oils, and fried foods. Skimmed or low-fat milk will give you all the nutrients you need with fewer calories. If you are thirsty, take extra fluid, but if you are overweight remember that nearly all drinks except water contain calories. Remember, too, that alcohol and caffeine pass through to your baby in your milk.

If you are still over your ideal weight by the time your baby is about six months old, reduce the quantity of your food intake while maintaining its quality and balance. Record your weight regularly (but not more than once a week) to ensure you are slowly losing excess fat. If you are breastfeeding, you should not attempt any crash diets as they may affect your health, energy, and milk supply. However, there is nothing to restrict the bottle-feeding mother from dieting sensibly from the start. Aerobic exercise – walking briskly, swimming, cycling, jogging – all help reduce excess body fat. If, despite adequate diet and rest, you feel excessively tired and irritable, you could be anemic and iron supplements may be prescribed by your doctor.

POSTURE AND BACK CARE

Your posture

Posture is the way you hold your body; it can often tell the world how you feel. If you are depressed or in pain you tend to slump.

What is good posture? It is not only a matter of appearance but also of function. It should be efficient, comfortable, and adaptable to the movements and positions used throughout the day. It is largely controlled by a reflex (subconscious) mechanism but is also considerably influenced by outside factors, such as emotions, neglected or damaged muscles, pain, and weight change. Fortunately, most postural faults can be corrected in a young, healthy person, but if they are not, they may go on to produce joint changes, sometimes leading to arthritis and long-term discomfort.

How pregnancy and birth influence posture

During pregnancy several factors contribute to an alteration in posture. Among these are the gradual increase in the size of your abdomen and in your weight, the softening of your ligaments (see page 12) and, possibly, the way you feel about your body and your pregnancy. As your baby and uterus grow, your center of gravity alters, which may cause you to lean back so that the hollow in your lumbar spine increases, your upper back rounds, and your chin pokes forward. Because your softer ligaments allow extra flexibility, your abdominal muscles will be forced to lengthen even more. If you are not aware that this is happening, your back muscles may shorten and extra stress will be placed on the ligaments and bones of your spine and pelvis. This change in posture causes backache. After your baby is born your body may be so used to this position that you have forgotten what your normal posture felt like. In addition, if you have pain in your perineum, breasts, or abdomen, or if you had a Caesarean section, you may sag forward as you shuffle along with your legs together, clutching your stomach. Holding an abnormal position because of pain, or the fear of it, is very tiring. You can be certain that your stitches are safe and that "standing tall," and taking a gentle walk, will improve not only your posture and appearance, but also your comfort.

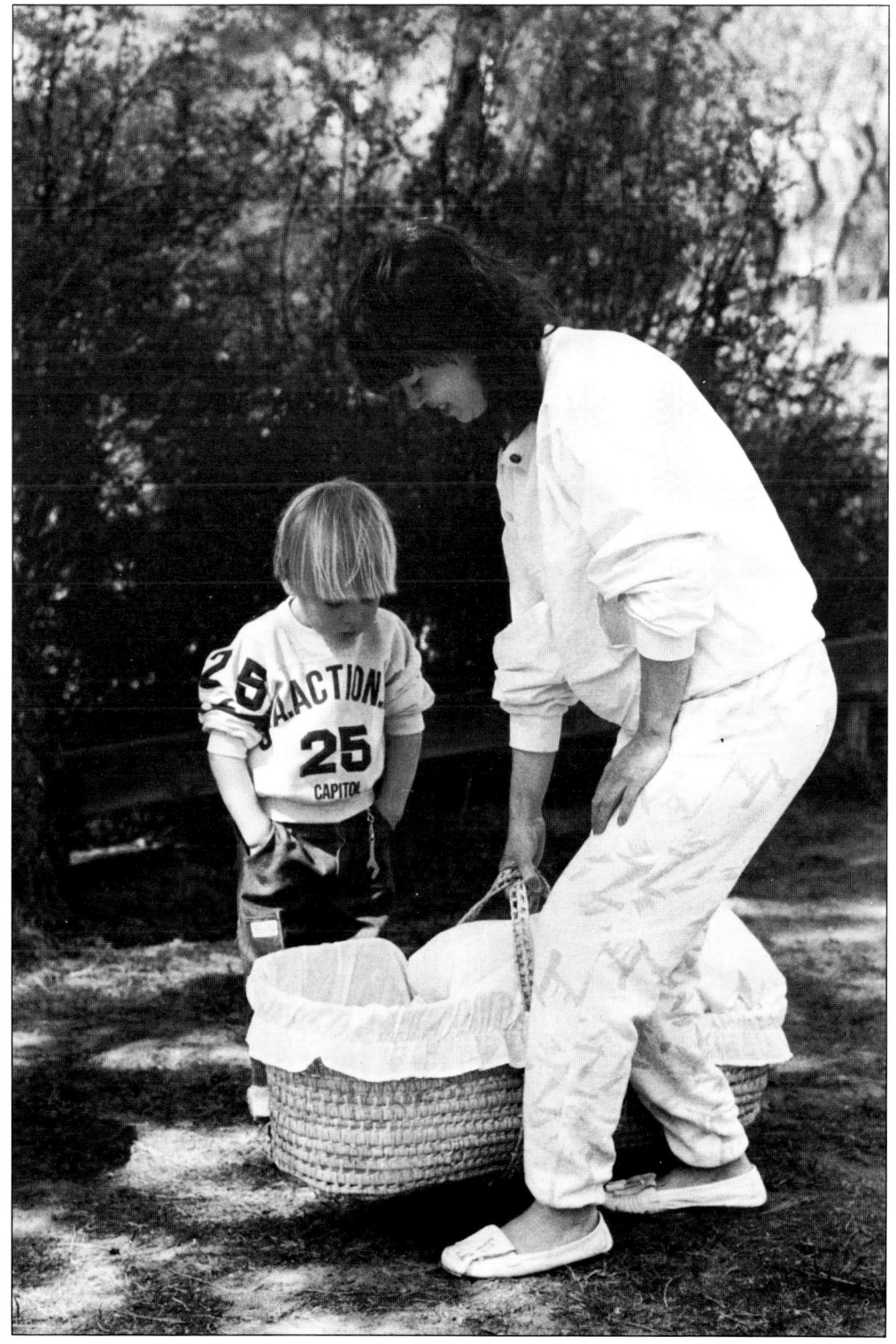

Correcting your posture

1 Look at yourself sideways in a long mirror, or ask a friend to check you. Stand as tall as you can: imagine someone is holding a tuft of hair from the top of your head and pulling it upward, making you taller.

2 Tuck your buttocks under and pull in your abdominal muscles as you tilt your whole pelvis backward so that your pubic bone moves forward and up. Lift your ribs away from your hips.

3 Move your feet about 12 in (30 cm) apart and feel the weight on their outside edges. Make sure your knees are relaxed and your arms hang loosely.

4 Relax your breathing to a slow, deep rhythm that is natural to you.

Feel your new posture. It may feel odd and unnatural at first, but be reassured by your mirror image or your critical friend that it has now improved.

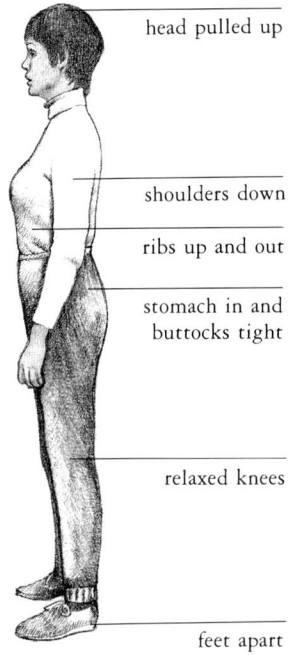

head pulled up

shoulders down

ribs up and out

stomach in and buttocks tight

relaxed knees

feet apart

Good posture

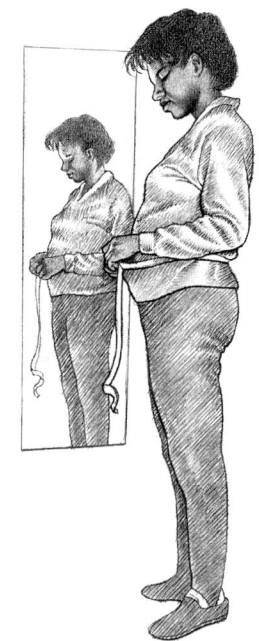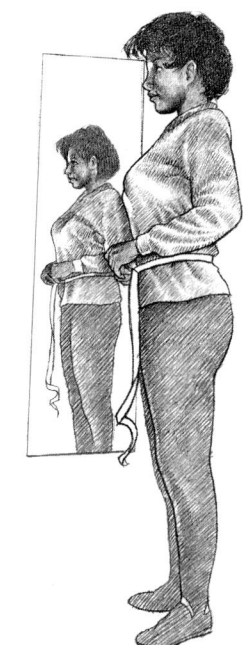

The tape measure test

The tape measure test

Pass a tape measure around the largest part of your abdomen and allow your body to sag. Then, lift your ribs, grow taller, tuck your bottom under and see the difference on the tape measure – good posture can make you 2–4 in (5–10 cm) thinner instantly!

Everyday back care

Because it can take five to six months for your ligaments to recover from the softening effects of the pregnancy hormones (see page 10), your spinal joints are more vulnerable to damage. Prevention is better than cure – be careful how you use your back.

Sitting

When you sit down, make sure you choose a chair that is the right height and depth, and that gives good support. The ideal chair has a firm back and a seat that provides support for your thighs while still allowing your knees to relax at right angles and your feet to rest flat on the floor. Tuck your bottom well into the back of the seat. You may find it even more comfortable to put a cushion behind your waist.

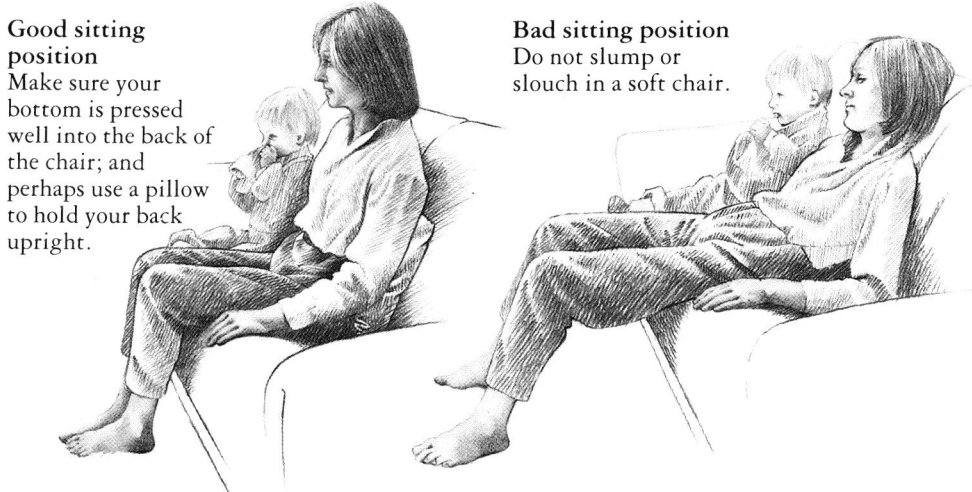

Good sitting position
Make sure your bottom is pressed well into the back of the chair; and perhaps use a pillow to hold your back upright.

Bad sitting position
Do not slump or slouch in a soft chair.

Lying

When you lie down to rest, make sure you are comfortable and that your vulnerable back is not strained and twisted in any way. If your bed is very soft, it will help if you slide a solid piece of plywood between the mattress and the bed base, or put the mattress on the floor so that it does not sag. If you like to lie on your back, try a pillow under your thighs to help flatten the hollow in your spine (see page 43).

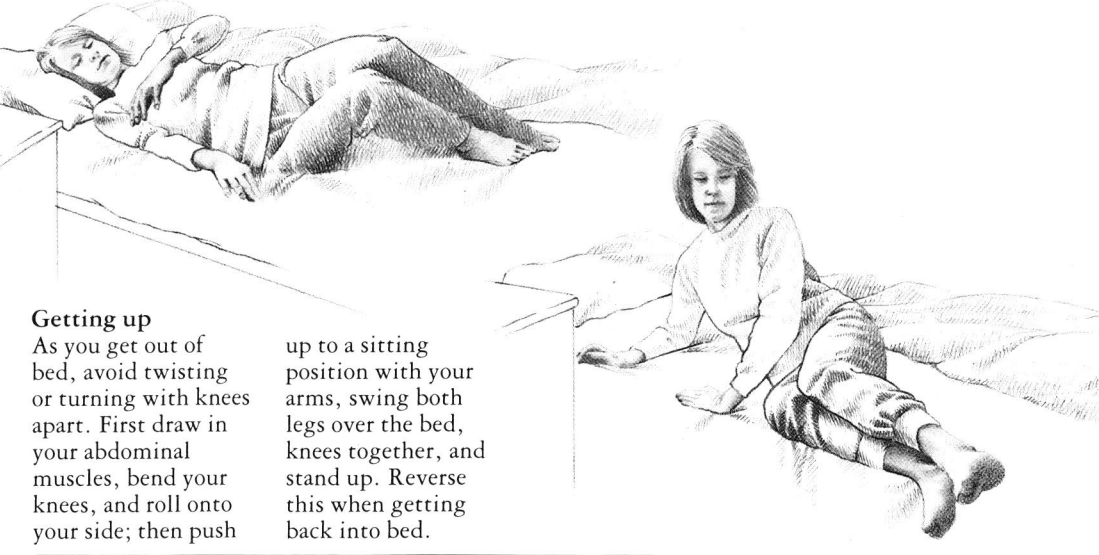

Getting up
As you get out of bed, avoid twisting or turning with knees apart. First draw in your abdominal muscles, bend your knees, and roll onto your side; then push up to a sitting position with your arms, swing both legs over the bed, knees together, and stand up. Reverse this when getting back into bed.

Lying on your front is an excellent position for relieving the pain of perineal stitches, hemorrhoids, and backache. Put one or even two pillows under your waist so that your back is flattened. You may find it more comfortable to have a pillow or two under your head and shoulders, so that your enlarged breasts are free from pressure. (If you have had a Caesarean section you will not be able to use this position immediately, but after two to three weeks you too will be able to enjoy it.) Rest in this position when you can. It has probably been impossible to lie on your stomach for months, so enjoy it now! Do be careful how you get up (see page 25).

Standing and working

When lifting anything heavy avoid twisting or bending your back to the side. Make sure your knees are bent and mobile if you have to push or pull a heavy weight, such as furniture. If you are lifting your baby in a bassinet, have the head nearest to you – this will put less strain on your back. Remember to protect your back by doing low household chores, such as making the bed or dressing your toddler, on your knees. Squat or kneel to pick things up off the floor. If you are vacuuming, move your weight forward and backward over your front leg, keeping your back straight; avoid twisting while bending forward.

Shoes can influence the way you stand. Flat or low heels lessen the tendency to hollow the back. It is important not to wear very high heels too often, as they will throw your weight even further forward and exaggerate the curve of your spine.

Lifting
When lifting a toddler or a heavy weight such as a full laundry basket, pull your abdominal

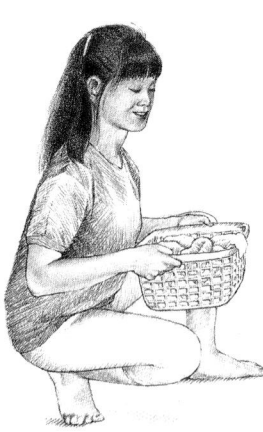

muscles in, tuck in your buttocks, and brace your pelvic floor. Keeping your back straight, bend your legs to kneel or squat down, bring the weight close to your body, and, using your stronger thighs to bear the weight, slowly rise to standing. This will protect the small muscles, ligaments, and joints of your spine and is also, incidentally, an excellent way of toning flabby thigh muscles. Never lift when bending or twisting to the side.

Standing
When you are standing to do household chores, put one foot up on a low stool or on two or three telephone directories, or rest one foot on the bottom shelf of a cupboard. This enables you to use your back more comfortably.

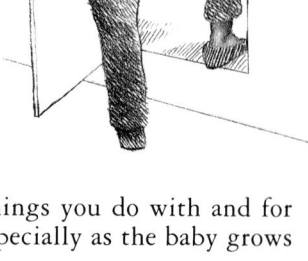

Back care and your baby

If you are not careful, many of the things you do with and for your baby can give you a backache, especially as the baby grows and becomes heavier.

Feeding

You will be spending many hours feeding your baby during the first few months; unsupported, sagging positions can make your back ache or increase any pain you may already have. Always make certain that you support your lower spine. Raising your baby by resting your feet on a low stool, a box, or a pile of books, and putting a pillow on your lap while your baby is small, can make the world of difference to your comfort.

If you prefer to feed sitting on the floor, make sure that your back is against a cupboard or wall.

Don't feed sitting on the edge of your bed so that your body sags forward. Instead sit well back against the bedhead with your back straight and well supported.

Breastfeeding while lying on your side is a very relaxing position and will help ease any backache you might have.

Good feeding position

Make sure your back is straight and well supported. Tuck a small, firm cushion behind your waist to support your lower spine. Lie your baby on a pillow and raise your feet by resting them on a low stool or a pile of books.

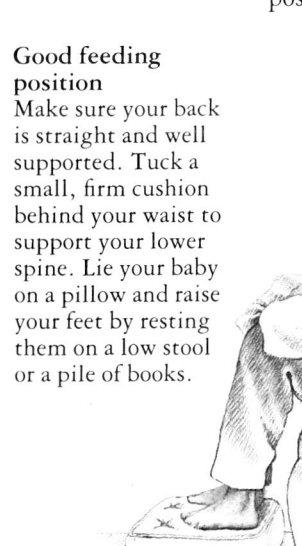

Bad feeding position
Don't sit unsupported, leaning forward.

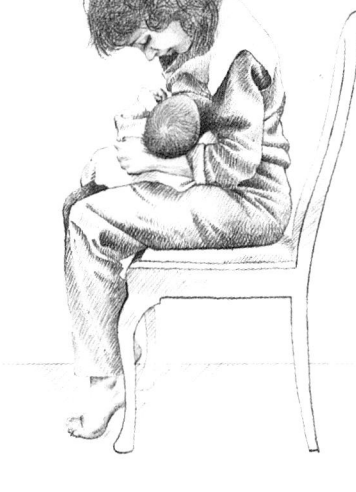

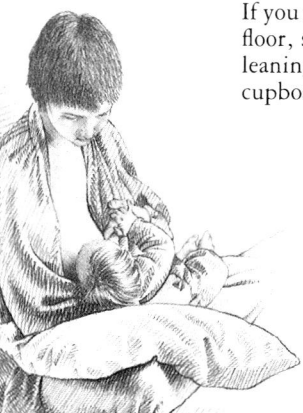

If you feed sitting on the floor, support your back by leaning against the wall or a cupboard.

Breastfeeding while lying on your side will help ease backache. Support your head on pillows and place one between your knees if that helps.

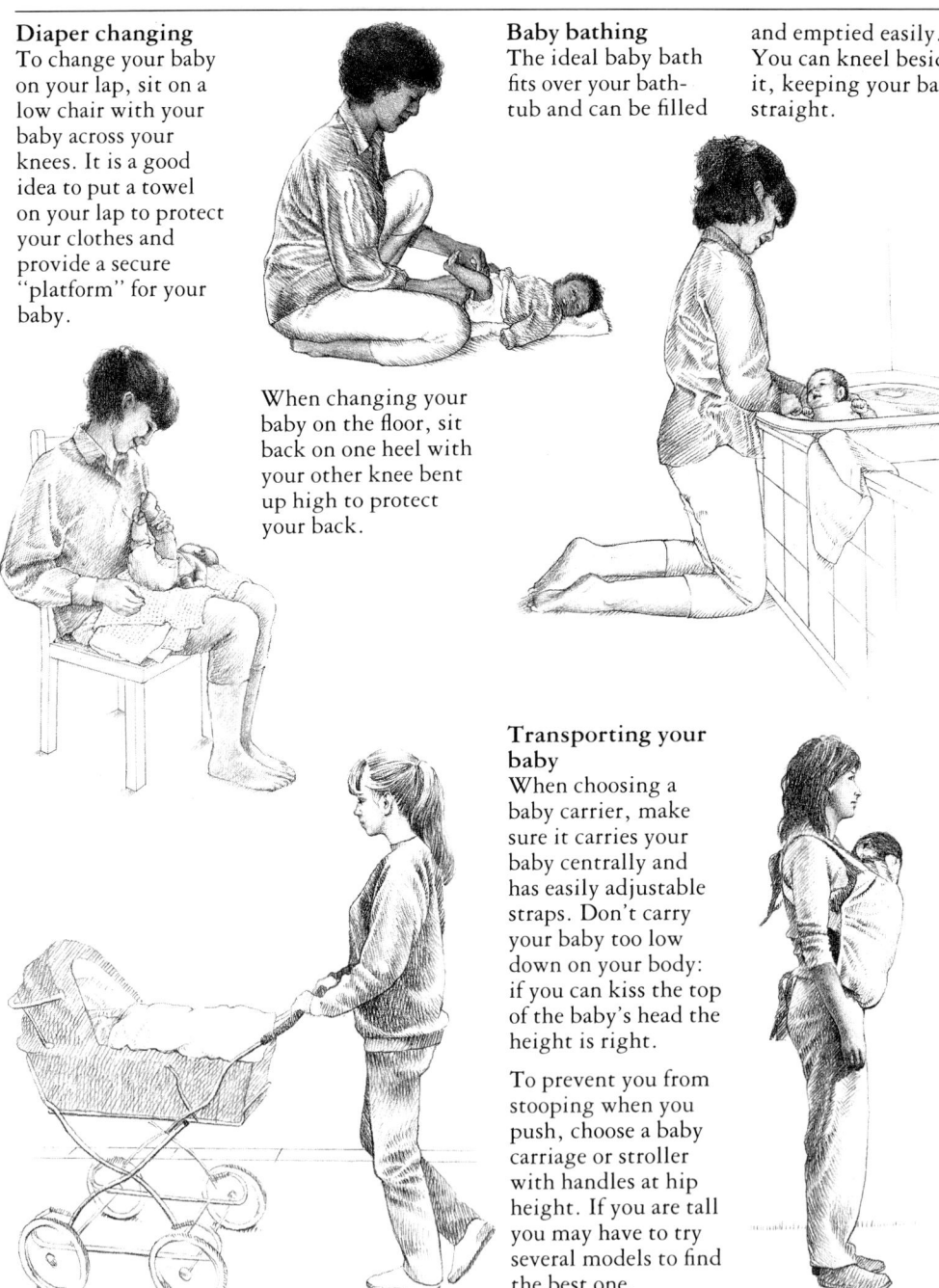

Diaper changing

To change your baby on your lap, sit on a low chair with your baby across your knees. It is a good idea to put a towel on your lap to protect your clothes and provide a secure "platform" for your baby.

When changing your baby on the floor, sit back on one heel with your other knee bent up high to protect your back.

Baby bathing

The ideal baby bath fits over your bath-tub and can be filled and emptied easily. You can kneel beside it, keeping your back straight.

Transporting your baby

When choosing a baby carrier, make sure it carries your baby centrally and has easily adjustable straps. Don't carry your baby too low down on your body: if you can kiss the top of the baby's head the height is right.

To prevent you from stooping when you push, choose a baby carriage or stroller with handles at hip height. If you are tall you may have to try several models to find the best one.

Diaper changing   You can change your baby while you sit, stand, or kneel, and it is most important to be careful because this is a job that can lead to back strain. Always have everything you need ready and within reach.

Sitting on a low chair with your baby across your lap is probably the best position for good back care. In the early months before your baby learns to roll, you may want to change her on a work top. Make sure it is at the right height – about waist level – so that you don't stoop. Changing your baby on the floor is an alternative but don't kneel and bend over him/her; make sure your back is as straight as possible by sitting back on one heel with your other knee bent up high. If you want to change your baby on your bed, do remember to kneel beside it. Don't stoop!

Baby bathing

Try to avoid baby baths on low stands that have to be filled with a pitcher or hose and emptied into a pail that you then have to lift and carry to the sink. Ideally, choose a bath that fits over your bathtub and that can be filled and emptied easily. Alternatively, bathe your new small baby in the bathroom sink or a large plastic tub on a table; as soon as he is a little bigger, he will enjoy being in the big bathtub, possibly with an older brother or sister.

Transporting your baby

When choosing a baby carrier, stroller, or carriage for carrying or transporting your baby, think of your back. Make sure a baby carrier can be easily adjusted (see page 65) so that your baby's head rests on your breastbone, just below your chin. Baby carriage or stroller handles should be hip height to prevent you from stooping when you push; some have adjustable handles that are useful if you and your partner are very different heights. You will, of course, need a rearward-facing car seat for the early months; it should be as light as possible with handles so it is easy to carry.

Backache and where it occurs

Postnatal back pain can occur anywhere in your spine from your neck to your coccyx. Neck and upper backache can be triggered by poor positions while breastfeeding, diaper changing, and baby bathing. Pain behind your waist may be the aftereffect of an epidural anesthetic, low back pain may be caused by ligaments stretching during labor and misuse of your back afterwards; and pain over your coccyx can result from it being pushed backward as your baby was born. Fatigue can also give rise or contribute to neck and backache.

A common site of pain after birth is the sacroiliac joint, where the spine joins the pelvis on either side (see page 12). It is normally felt over the joint (that lies immediately under one of the two dimples on either side of the spine). The pain may radiate into the whole buttock, and there is sometimes associated tenderness at the front over the pubic bone. The backache experienced can be constant, and there may be pain down the leg. Walking short distances is often reasonably comfortable, but the pain will then usually get progressively worse. It may be difficult to bear weight on the affected leg (such as when climbing stairs), there is little relief felt after lying down, and you may feel stiff after a period of sitting. Turning over in bed can also be painful.

Intervertebral disc damage

Very severe pain may be caused by damage to a disc between the vertebrae of the spine. It may cause lumbago (incapacitating pain in the lower back) or sciatica (pain along the sciatic nerve – through the buttock, back of the thigh and calf, and into the foot); the pain will be most severe when sitting, coughing, and bending forward – which will be restricted. Lying down often relieves the symptoms. The treatment for severe disc problems is usually bed rest. If this fails to help relieve your pain, see your doctor.

RELIEVING BACK PAIN

You may have followed the advice on how to protect your back, but if you experience backache, there are several ways to alleviate and often ease it.

Upper or thoracic back pain can often be eased by shoulder-circling (see page 45) and neckache can be soothed by turning your head first to one side and then the other.

Reverse pelvic thrusts lying on your back (see page 51), lying on your side (Side-lying Curls, page 50), sitting on a chair (Sitting Pelvic Rocks, page 56), and standing up (Standing Pelvic Rocks, page 59) – all are excellent for relieving backache associated with fatigue and tension.

If your pain is localized to the sacroiliac joints, lie on the floor and try one or both of the following exercises. When doing them, use the leg on the side of the body that is painful. The illustration for the first exercise (below) shows how to obtain relief for pain on the right side. Relieving pain on the left side is illustrated in the second exercise.

FLEXED KNEE STRETCHES
Relief for right-sided pain is illustrated. Bend your right leg up, holding it around the knee with your right hand, and with your left hand pull your right heel toward your groin. Keeping your shoulders flat and left leg straight, press the bent leg farther up toward the right shoulder, as far as it will comfortably go, then relax. Press and relax several times, then, get up: keeping your knees bent and together, roll onto your side, push up onto all fours, and stand carefully, keeping your back straight.

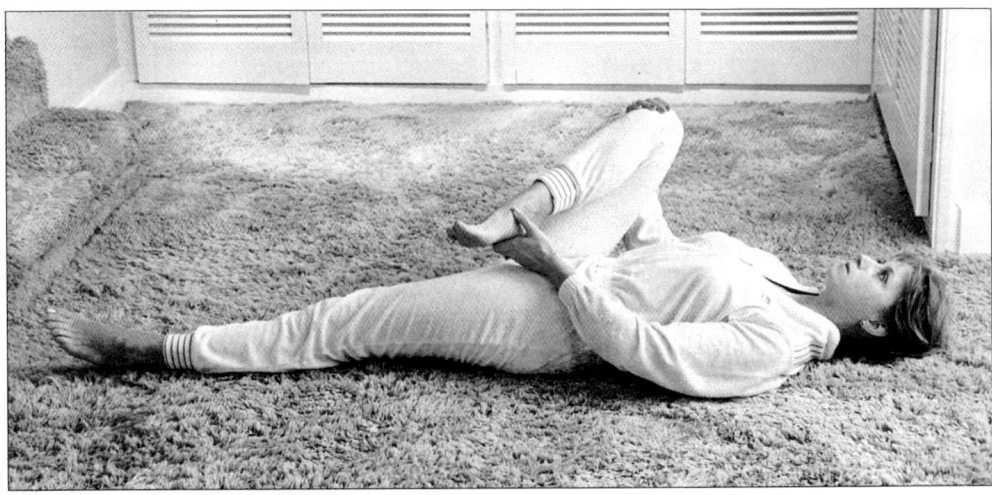

LATERAL TWISTS

Lie on your back on the floor. For left-sided pain, bend your left leg and hook your toes under the outside of your right calf and roll your left knee toward the right. Now take your right arm across your body so that your hand holds your left hip. Rock gently in this position; then roll back to the starting position and relax. Repeat several times. Again take care when you stand up – knees together to roll onto your side, then push onto all fours, and keep your back straight as you rise to stand.

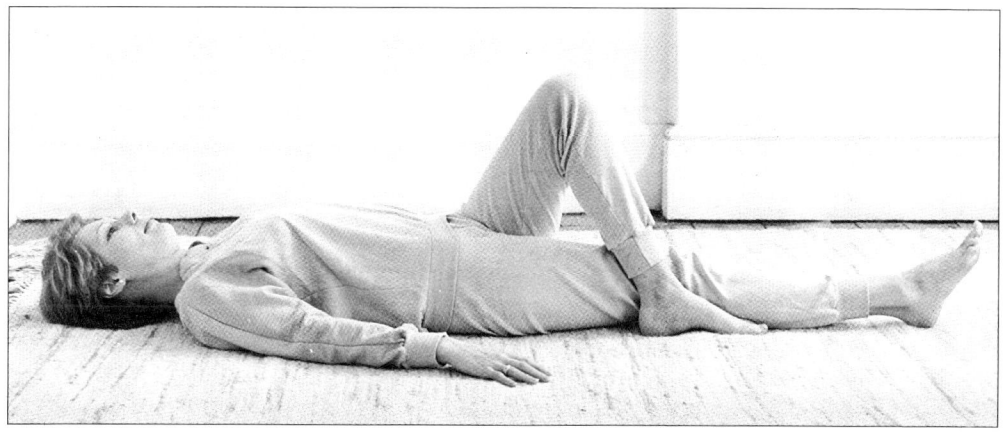

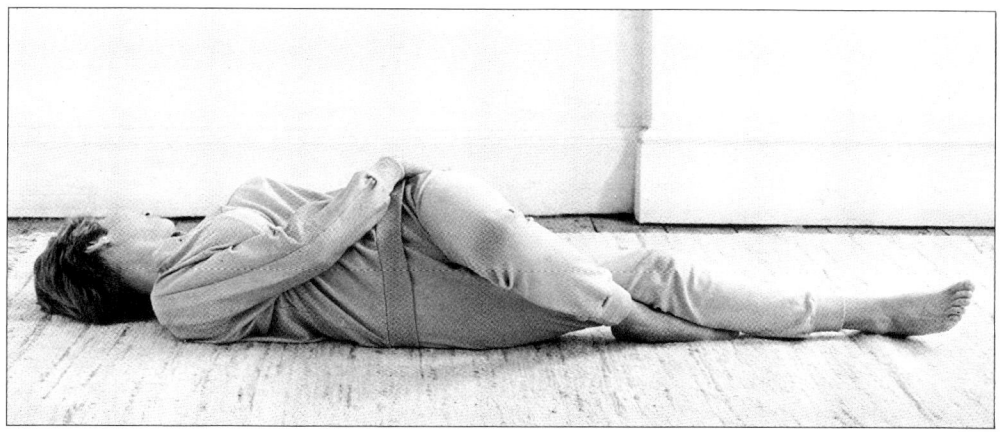

Taking medical advice

If low back pain continues, as a first aid measure try wearing a pantie girdle to support the aching joints. It may give very good relief and will not weaken your abdominal muscles as long as you remember to exercise them and use them to hold yourself in.

If your backache begins to affect your ability to cope with your family, then do not hesitate to seek medical advice. Treatment may be simple, or you may be advised to take a period of rest in bed. Whatever is needed, you must try to tackle the problem now, however inconvenient or impossible it may seem. Back problems have a habit of recurring as acute and crippling episodes or chronic, nagging aches.

YOUR FEELINGS
AFTER THE BIRTH

Emotional changes

No matter how intensely you looked forward to the birth of your baby, or how much you expected that the rewards of motherhood would compensate for your loss of freedom or job satisfaction, it is as well to be prepared for a tiring, tense, and possibly traumatic first few weeks. Women change and develop emotionally as much as physically during the early days of motherhood.

In the same way that the enlarging uterus and softening ligaments of pregnancy trouble some women during the gestation of their babies – so the change in life-style from independence to motherhood can also prove painful for some. In fact, becoming a parent is one of life's most important revolutions, and is often described as a "life crisis," similar to the upheaval involved in marriage, bereavement, changing or losing a job, or moving house. However, if you are prepared for some of the feelings and problems that can occur after your baby is born, you may be able to cope with them more easily.

Immediate feelings after the birth

The way you feel in the first few hours following delivery can vary enormously. You may be euphoric, flat, detached, tearful, overjoyed, or disappointed. Alot will depend on the length and type of labor you have just experienced. Naturally you are going to feel more tired if your labor has been long and painful, especially if you missed out on more than one night's sleep. You may have set yourself all sorts of goals to achieve in labor, and feel like a failure because, instead of an active, natural childbirth, you ended up with painkillers, an epidural, an episiotomy, and a forceps delivery. You may have set your heart on a golden-haired daughter and have gotten instead a dark-haired son with forceps marks on his face, who looks like your least favorite relative. Some women fall in love with their babies instantly, but many others have a detached feeling about them – their overriding reaction being a desire to roll over and go to sleep.

Apart from the initial fatigue that follows labor, tremendous changes in the hormonal balance may also affect the emotions.

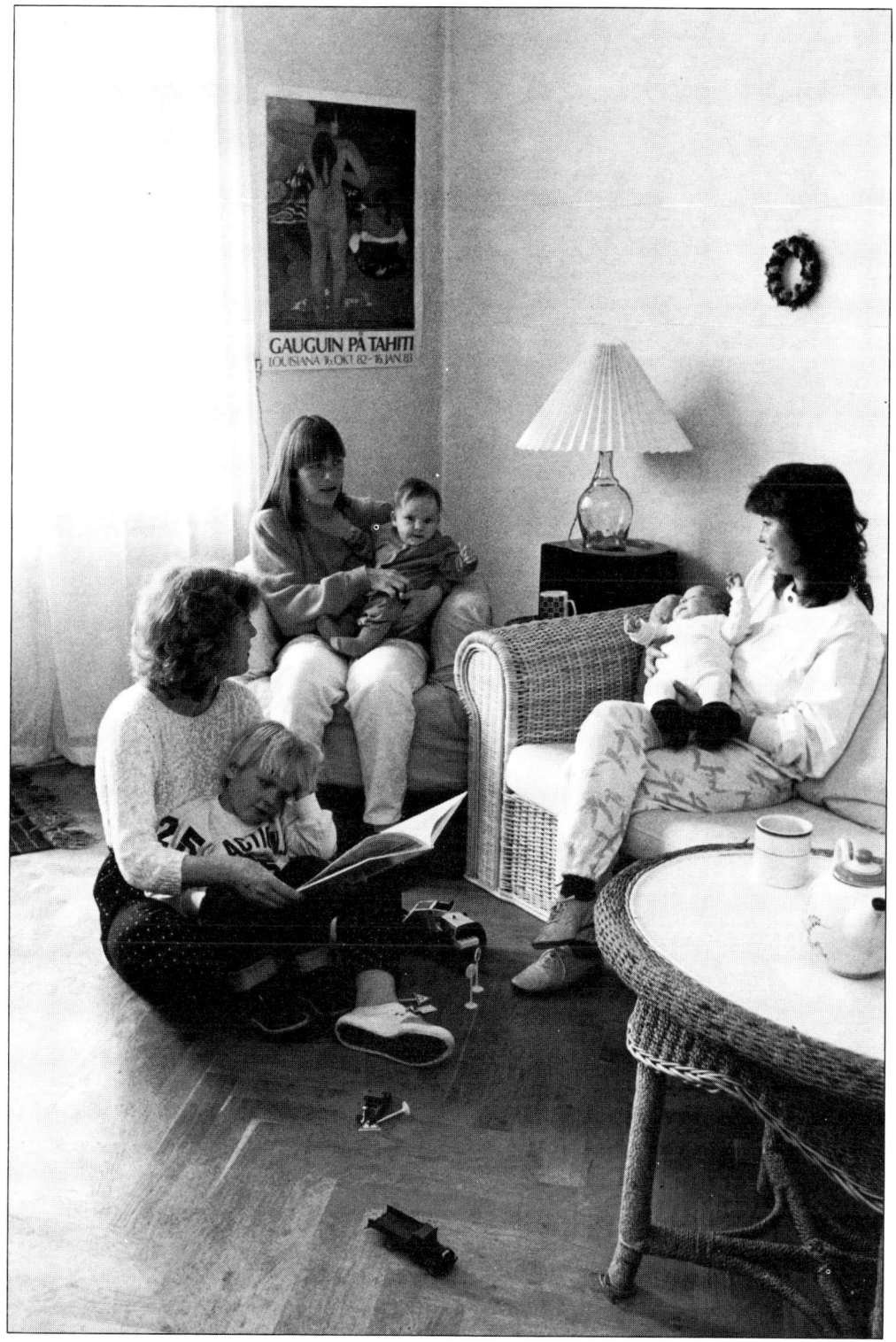

The hormones that have been controlling the pregnancy are replaced by those that stimulate the breasts to produce milk, and return the body to its pre-pregnant state. These changes may cause overwhelming shifts in mood.

Something you may not have been expecting is missing the presence of your baby within your body. Even though you have been longing for your balloonlike shape to disappear, you may feel empty and lonely after your baby is born and miss his movements intensely; your baby will almost certainly feel lonely too. Another strange and probably completely unexpected feeling is a sense of anticlimax. Labor, which is often seen as the "grand finale" of pregnancy before you return to normal, is actually the "overture" to a completely new life-style.

Baby blues

"Baby blues" is a common and distressing reaction. It usually creeps up on you between two days and a week after the birth, or even later. Emotions that go up have to come down. If the first 48 hours of your role as mother has floated by in a haze of pink cloud, it can be a shock then to experience tearfulness, depression, and feelings of anxiety and helplessness. Little things may trigger bouts of crying – maybe your partner arrives five minutes late for visiting time; or a nurse speaks to you abruptly. You may also notice violent mood swings, one minute feeling intense surges of mother love, the next being driven to desperation because the baby is crying. It may help you to know that well over 50 percent of all mothers suffer from this temporary problem.

First days at home

Once you are home with your baby the most devastating discovery for the first-time mother may be that you are on duty 24 hours a day, every day – there is no letup. First-timers have the additional burden of having to learn how to be mothers and fathers; parents having a subsequent baby have learned this lesson and birth is probably not such an overwhelming experience, although the existing family has to adapt to the new baby.

Many women who had responsible jobs feel like failures because they cannot cope domestically – the chores pile up and they are still in their bathrobes by mid-afternoon. You may feel like a failure if you cannot establish breastfeeding, but bottle-feeding too can present problems.

Catching up with sleep

Most young women are used to an uninterrupted night's sleep of eight to nine hours, and it can take several months to get used to your new way of life and for the intense fatigue to disappear. Your motto at first should be, "sleep when the baby sleeps," which is easy after a first baby, but not quite so easy if you already have older children. If you cannot fit in an hour or two of sleep during the day, make the most of little "catnaps" whenever you can. Rest and relax – using the simple relaxation drill on page 40, and make sure that feeding times are restful and relaxing too: put your feet up or curl up on your side on your bed. Make up your mind that for a while you do not need a spotlessly clean house; this is something that your partner can help with. If cooking is a problem for both of you, convenience foods or take-out meals are worth the extra expense for a while.

Finally, there will be days when rest is more important to you than exercises. Don't worry if you are unable to fit the exercises in every day, and don't exercise at 11.30 at night when you are dropping with fatigue.

Crisis measure

If you feel that you are so drained of energy you cannot go on any longer, a useful tip is to go to bed as soon as you have eaten dinner – say at 7 pm – and sleep until your baby wakes for a feeding. Ask your partner to bring the baby to you in bed; let him change the diaper– if necessary – halfway through the feeding; then, when your baby is full of food and drops off to sleep, do the same, until the next feeding.

Anxiety and stress

Anxiety is an emotion that may constantly plague you during those early weeks; feeding, changing, sleeping all seem fraught with uncertainties. You may reach the stage when you feel compelled to telephone your partner, begging him to come home and relieve you. He is your link with the outside world and you need his support. Some parents try to continue their lives as if nothing had happened, determined that the baby should in no way alter their cozy twosome – but it is practically impossible initially to be a perfect mother, partner, and lover simultaneously.

Your relationship with your partner

First-time childbirth often disrupts a relationship in a way that can be totally unexpected – after all, a twosome that increases by 50 percent to become a threesome is no longer the same, and there is bound to be a period of adjustment before the new situation is accepted. You may find you feel very dependent, and this need for support will continue for a time after the birth. You will be constantly preoccupied with the baby, certainly very tired and anxious, and possibly depressed too, and you may be unable to give your partner the care and attention he wants. You may find you both have unspoken fears about sex; you may not feel desire for a while; he may be frightened of hurting you.

If you both decide before the birth that initially it will be your partner's job to care for you both by taking on as much of the shopping, cooking, and cleaning as he can manage, the early weeks will be much easier for all of you, and your relationship with each other will become much more of a partnership and therefore much more serene; whereas, if you desperately try to cope with everything *and* the baby, relations can be strained. Either way, fathers need to be involved from the beginning and communication is the key, so try and talk it through.

The older child

Another relationship that may change following the birth of a new baby is the one you have with your older children. Many parents worry and feel guilty before the birth of a second baby, particularly if there is a small age gap between the two children. When the baby arrives they feel that perhaps they are being

35

unfair to their firstborn, displacing him while he is still a baby.

Toddlers may show their jealousy by reverting to babyish habits – waking at night and forgetting their toilet training. They may not show their animosity to the baby directly, but will become "difficult" in their attempts to capture *your* interest. Even if there is a gap of many years, older children can show their anxiety and fear of being displaced in your affection by becoming truculent and untidy. It is difficult for firstborn children to appreciate that all children in a family are loved, and only time, plus your continued reassurance, will show them that they mean as much to you as their rival. Of course life has to continue, and chores have to be done – but many early relationship problems can happily be dealt with by touching and cuddling and *showing* each other that, although the pattern of interaction has changed, affection and love are still there.

Preventing loneliness

Loneliness may be something you never experienced before your first baby was born. It is not until you are actually home – alone with your baby – that you might suddenly feel very isolated and miss adult conversation and company.

To avoid this, it is a good idea to exchange telephone numbers with some of the other expectant mothers in your prenatal class, so that even if you are the first among your own friends or family to have a baby you will still be able to communicate with someone who appreciates how difficult those early weeks can be. The telephone can be a lifeline, even though it is not the same as human company.

Ask your doctor if he or she knows of someone who has recently had a baby and who lives nearby; start conversations with other mothers when you visit the pediatrician, and ask if they have a "Mother and Baby Club." La Leche League has postnatal support groups, and many childbirth education groups sponsor mother-to-mother and mother-baby discussion sessions. It might be helpful if you tell yourself that you are not the only new mother who is feeling so alone, and that probably most of the women you see in the supermarket and in the street with tiny babies are feeling the same way.

Postnatal depression

Most women will pass safely through the postnatal period with nothing more than a mild attack of the blues to bother them. However, for 10 percent or so, a more severe form of emotional upset – postnatal depression – can become a long-lasting, trying condition. It does not necessarily begin immediately after the baby is born; indeed, it may be several weeks or months before it occurs, but its effect on both mother and family is shattering.

Symptoms of depression

Most postnatally depressed women complain of extreme exhaustion – not just the normal postnatal fatigue but something much more intense and continuous. Sadness and weepiness, a sense of inadequacy, tension, and anxiety, irrational fears – these are all symptoms of this very common disorder. Some women complain of physical symptoms too – palpitations, dizziness, aching all over, an inability to sleep in spite of their tiredness, or a complete loss of libido (sexual interest). Sometimes a woman will complain of loss of appetite and will lose weight; yet other women will feel the need to go on frequent eating binges, putting on excessive weight instead of losing it. Women suffering from postnatal depression are often unsmiling, very irritable, short-tempered, and can experience terrifying moments when they really hate their children and desperately want to hurt them.

Feelings of aggression

You may have thought that your baby would sleep for 20 hours each day, only waking every so often for a feeding, so that you would have plenty of time for yourself. It is quite a shock to realize that even a two-week-old baby can stay awake for hours on end needing constant entertainment, driving you, meanwhile, to distraction. All normal parents will admit to terrifying moments when their baby pushes them to the brink of violence. Thankfully, most of us step back from this, horrified by our feelings. Try not to feel too guilty about them; instead learn to recognize the signs, counter them with the crisis relaxation techniques given later on page 42, and find someone sympathetic in whom you can confide (Useful Addresses, see page 125).

Dealing with depression

It is useless to tell a depressed woman to "pull herself together" – she cannot do it. At a time when she feels she should be glowing with happiness and contentment, enjoying her new baby and family and coping with all the domestic chores as efficiently and easily as before her pregnancy, she finds herself in a state of despondency and hopelessness.

Fortunately, postnatal depression is now recognized much more frequently by doctors – and by mothers and their families too. It can be treated and women can be helped over this distressing period. Psychotherapy and/or antidepressant pills are used with good results. If you are still breastfeeding, your doctor will take this into account and only prescribe treatment that is safe for the baby. Talking to people about your feelings can help enormously – your family, doctor, other women in the clinic, friends with older children. They will all understand and will help you realize that emotional illness can be a part of childbirth for some women, and, for the vast majority of them, can be dealt with swiftly leading to complete recovery.

Getting back to normal

The passing of time soon brings its compensations. The early weeks of constant caring gradually change when you see that first dazzling smile, when your baby "talks" back to you, and follows your movements around the room. Suddenly your baby is beginning to learn to socialize and you realize that normal life goes on outside the confines of parenthood, and there will be moments that you will treasure and that will remain with you even when your "baby" has grown into an adult who has begun to earn his or her own living!

At the end of the first three months the continuous hard physical work of caring for a new baby begins to be worth it – and both you and your partner will be glad to be parents after all.

THE IMPORTANCE
OF RELAXATION

During pregnancy your preparation for labor may have included learning relaxation techniques that help the body to cope with stress and work more efficiently. Even if you produce a large family, the total number of hours spent in labor during a lifetime is tiny, but the relaxation techniques learned in your prenatal classes can be applied to your life in general, and especially to those early days and weeks following birth.

Babies are born knowing instinctively how to relax; you will feel your own baby's deep relaxation when you hold him or her close to your body. Your body knows how to relax too; every night when you drift into sleep the muscles of your body stop working and relax. Even without sleep you know how to relax; when you lie on the beach or in your backyard, soaking up the summer sun, your body comfortably supported, your muscles have no need to work and they relax. Faced with a stressful situation, however, you become tense – and your body will always react in the same way, regardless of the cause. Even babies respond to stress – pain, discomfort, loneliness, the fear of being dropped, or anger at not being fed.

The effects of stress

The stresses and strains we experience as we pass through childhood and adolescence to reach adult life produce tensions in the muscles that can give rise to postural distortions: raised tense shoulders, clenched fists, jaws clamped tightly together, pressed lips, furrowed forehead, and altered respiration. Mental turmoil often leads to physical tension and the vicious circle is established: the body reacts to the anxieties felt within by hunching, clenching, tightening muscles, and gritting teeth; this leads to aches and pains and more emotional distress. This reaction to stress is one of your body's primitive reflexes. You sense danger, and at once your muscles tense, ready to fight or run away. Other responses include sweating, pallor, pounding heart, dry mouth, and faster, deeper respiration.

During pregnancy, the prospect of labor and delivery stand

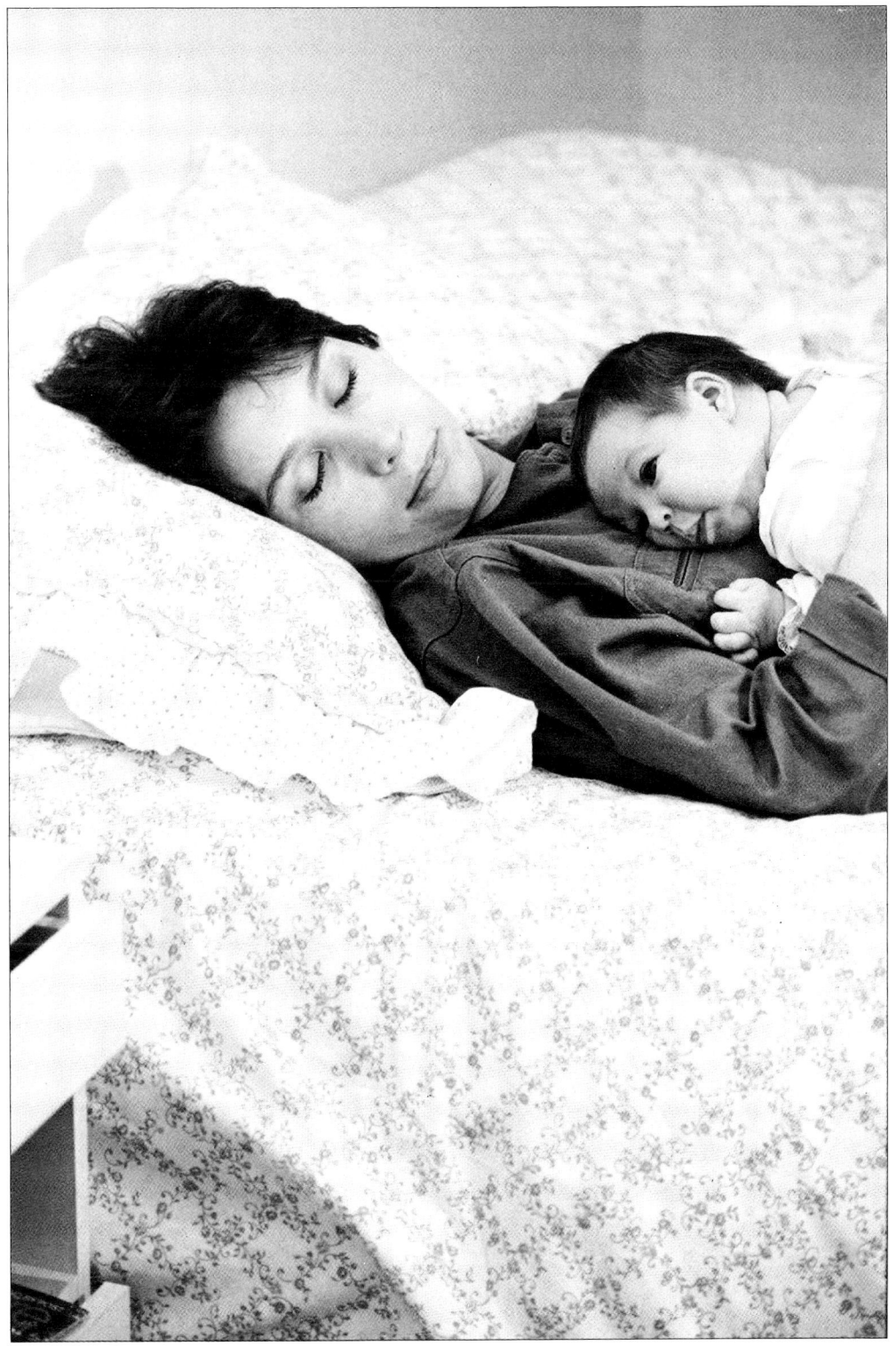

before you rather like the highest mountain of a range; once you have climbed it and reached its peak (the moment of birth) you imagine that the descent to new parenthood will be easy. As we have seen, you may in fact be totally unprepared for the reality of the early days and weeks of your new baby's life. Tension and fatigue seem to increase hourly; when your baby wakes for the fourth time one night, your body reacts by producing the primitive stress response. You try to pacify him with tight, raised shoulders, anxiety and tiredness wrinkling your face – and a coiled spring of tension within you that may make you want to shake the poor child back to sleep.

Reciprocal relaxation

Fortunately, there is a very useful law of the body called "reciprocal relaxation" that can help you move away from the tense, hunched posture invoked by stress. While one group of muscles works to perform a movement, the opposite group has to relax. This is a physiological fact that you can use to help yourself. For example, to bring ease and comfort to tightly clenched teeth, you can work the muscles that oppose the upward pull on your jaw. Try this: clench your teeth. Then, with your lips together, drag the lower jaw down – stop doing it and then notice the new position of your teeth, slightly apart. Your jaws are now relaxed.

"Physiological relaxation"

Picture your reaction to the extreme stress of fear. Your shoulders are up, arms pulled into your sides, elbows bent, and hands clenched, legs ready to run, body crouched forward, chin tucked into your chest, your face distorted. The following sequence of movements – a technique known as "physiological relaxation" – is the direct opposite to those your body makes to achieve the tension posture. Because of the law of reciprocal relaxation, following each individual movement tense parts of your body will *always* become relaxed. Bit by bit you can take your body away from the posture of tension to the position of ease, comfort, and relaxation.

Practicing "physiological relaxation"

Lie down comfortably on your back with your head and thighs supported by pillows.

1 **Shoulders** Pull your shoulders toward your feet – then stop pulling. Register the new position of ease in your mind – your shoulders are relaxed.

2 **Arms** Push your elbows out and open – stop pushing when you feel your position to be comfortable; register this position – your arms are relaxed.

3 **Hands** Let them rest comfortably on your thighs or abdomen. Stretch the fingers so that they are long and straight; stop. Notice their new position – loosely curled and relaxed.

4 **Hips** Tighten your buttocks and press your knees out sideways. Stop doing it – notice the relaxed sensation in your hips.

5 **Knees** Lift your heels; stop doing it – and register the comfortable feeling in your knees and thighs.

6 **Feet** Press your feet away from your face. Stop doing it – and notice comfortable feet dangling on the ends of your legs.

7 **Body** Press your body into the support behind you; stop doing it – and register the pleasant sensation of relaxation in your abdomen.

8 **Head** Press your head into the support behind it – stop pressing – and notice how this movement has relaxed your neck and upper shoulders. (If you want to try this while sitting in a chair and your head is not supported, let it tilt forward slightly till it reaches a comfortable position.)

9 **Face** (a) your jaw: drag your lower jaw down; stop doing it – then notice the pleasant feeling of comfort that you have when your upper and lower sets of teeth are resting slightly apart.

(b) your mouth: stretch your lips sideways in a little smile, pout your lips forward very quickly and then notice the pleasing sensation of soft, warm lips just lightly touching each other.

(c) your eyes: your lids are resting comfortably over your eyes. You may even want to close them.

(d) your forehead: imagine that someone is stroking it and smoothing away the lines of tension.

Relaxing your jaw
Clenched teeth (right) often accompany tension. Drag your jaw down keeping your lips touching (center); then stop and let your teeth rest slightly apart (far right).

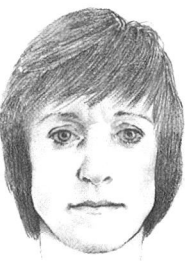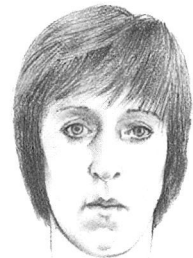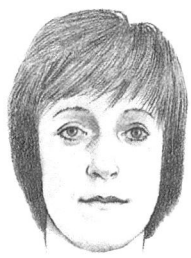

Breathing for relaxation

Because the way you breathe is affected by stress, altering your respiration is one of the easiest ways of inducing relaxation. You tend to breathe out as you relax: imagine your reaction to finding a purse that you'd thought you'd lost – with next week's food money in it – you sigh with relief and relax. If you use this response to deal with the many problems that crop up continuously during parenthood, they can often be resolved painlessly. Breathe out and relax at the beginning of a feeding if you feel the needlelike pain from a sore nipple. Breathe out and relax when you realize that you have run out of diapers. Breathe out and relax when your toddler unravels a completely new roll of toilet paper or empties the contents of his potty on the floor.

Use your breathing to increase the depth of your relaxation. Make it slow, calm, and quiet. Concentrate on the outward breath – empty your chest – pause – and then let only as much air into your lungs as you need at that particular moment – do not force more and more air into your chest.

The beauty of the relaxation technique is that it always works, day or night, whatever your position and whatever you are doing (washing, feeding the baby, waiting for a bus). It is not always necessary to lie down in a darkened room surrounded by silence to be able to relax. You can take your hunched shoulders away from their tense position by simply moving them in the opposite direction.

Using the relaxation technique It is not necessary to run through all the movements every time. Your shoulders, arms, hands, and face are usually the first parts of your body to respond to stress – recognize the tension in them and release it by adjusting the stress-induced posture.

Whenever your baby is sleeping, experiment with comfortable positions in which you can rest, doze, or sleep yourself. Feeding time gives you a wonderful opportunity to practice relaxation, for tension is catching; if you start nursing your baby while sitting uncomfortably, your back will begin to ache, you may be scared to move in case your baby stops sucking, you will become tense and long for the feeding ,to be over. In turn, your baby may sense this and will become disturbed and restless. Anxiety at the beginning of a feeding can delay the "let down" reflex that makes the milk-producing glands release the milk in your breasts. Use your relaxation to overcome this. Always make sure you are comfortable, close your eyes (if it helps), and consciously run through the body movements to give you total relaxation.

Many mothers find it hard to get back to sleep once they have been disturbed by their baby at night. Use your relaxation technique and slow calm breathing to help you float into sleep again. Relaxation is a valuable tool, always there for you to use during crises. Remember, by practicing this useful technique, you will be *using* time and not wasting it, and it will become a lifelong legacy of childbirth.

Crisis measures When you reach the breaking point, try this emergency relaxation. Breathe out – then, breathing naturally:

Face Smooth away worry lines – teeth apart.

Shoulders Down – stop – feel it.

Hands Long stretched fingers – stop – feel it.

Comfortable relaxation or resting positions

It is helpful to relax for five to ten minutes after you have completed your daily postnatal exercise sessions. The positions suggested in the Daily Programs (pages 62, 89, and 112) are only given as guides; you could use whichever position described here seems most comfortable at the time.

Sit at a table with your knees wide apart and feet flat on the floor, resting your head on your arms.

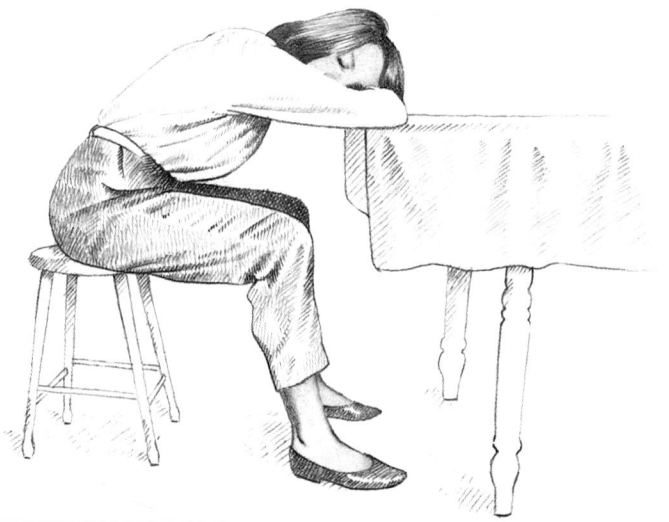

Lie on your front with a pillow or two under your hips and abdomen and another one or two under your head and shoulders to take the weight off your breasts. This position is particularly useful for the immediate postnatal period when you may have an uncomfortable perineum, hemorrhoids, or back.

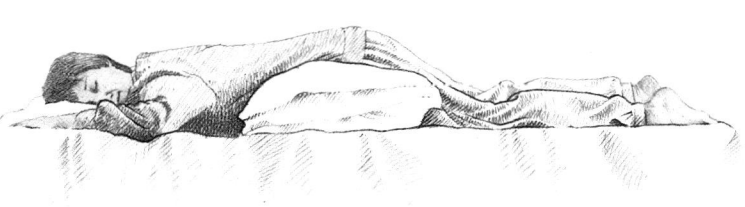

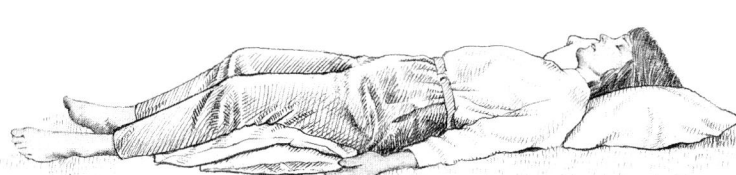

Lie flat on your back with legs apart and palms up. Support your head with pillows and place another under your thighs.

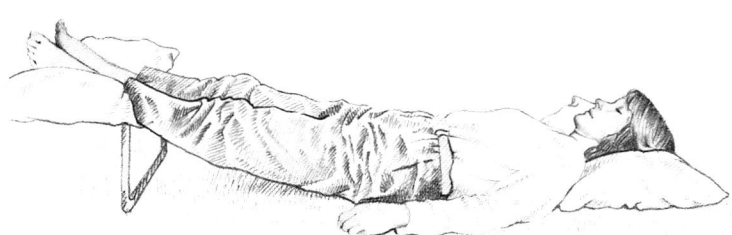

An alternative to the above position is to raise your legs by resting your feet on a low stool or coffee table, with one pillow placed under your heels and another under your head.

If you are comfortable sitting back on your heels, you can relax while resting your head on a firm sofa cushion. Make sure that your knees are wide apart, and your arms well forward so that you can also enjoy the feeling of 'stretch' in your back.

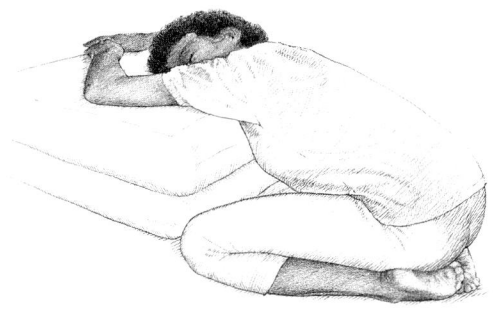

EASY RELAXATION EXERCISES

UNCURLING

Stand up and bend forward so that your shoulders and arms hang heavily. Stay there, resting and breathing quietly. Slowly uncurl, bringing your body upward. When you are straight, stand still for a moment, breathing quietly. You may like to arch your back, supporting your waist with your hands. You can also do this exercise sitting in a chair with your knees wide apart.

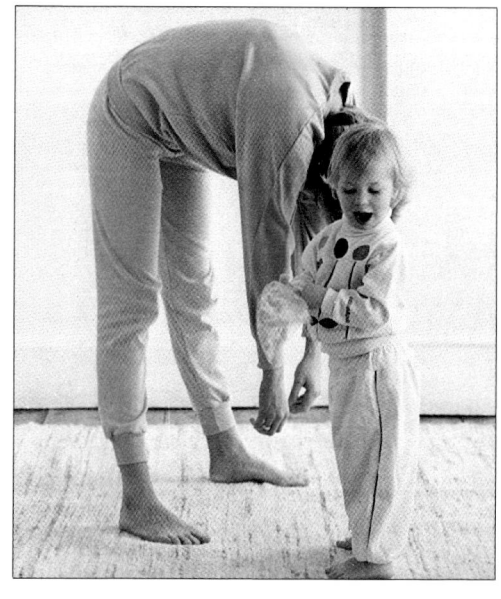

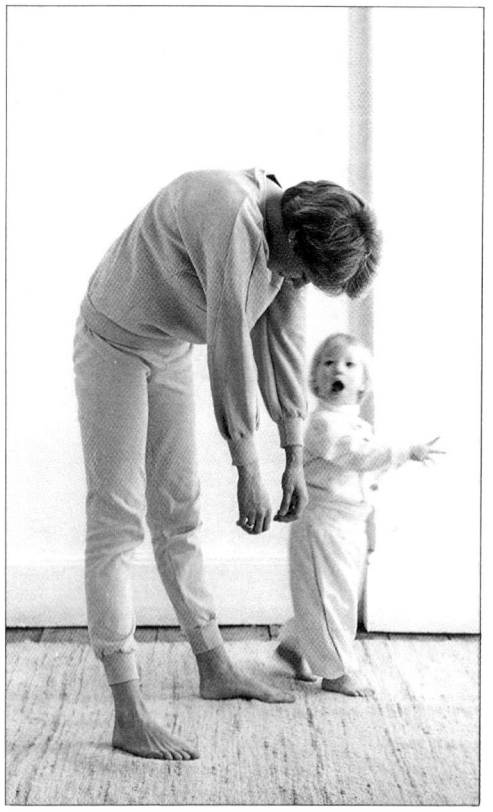

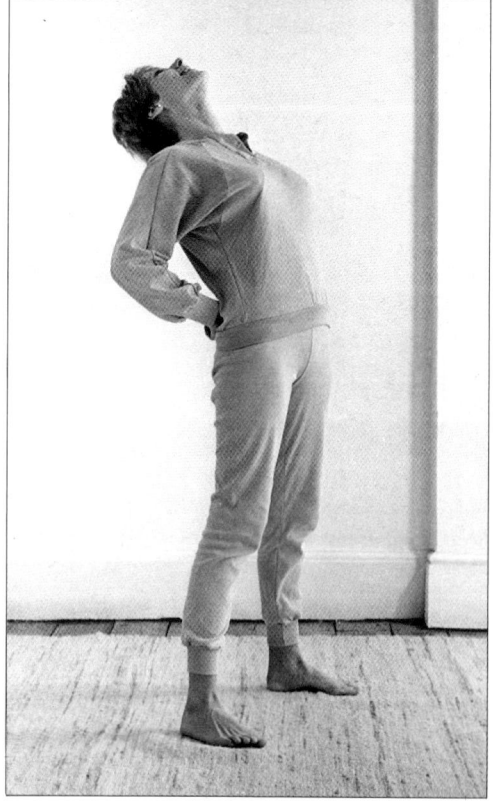

SHOULDER-CIRCLING

Circle your shoulders backward, first one, then the other and then both together several times. Finish with them both down in a relaxed position. This relieves neck and shoulder tension.

ARM-STRETCHING

S-T-R-E-T-C-H your arms as high as you can above your head; then stop and bring them down and relax. You can do this stretching movement sitting down, standing up, or lying on your bed.

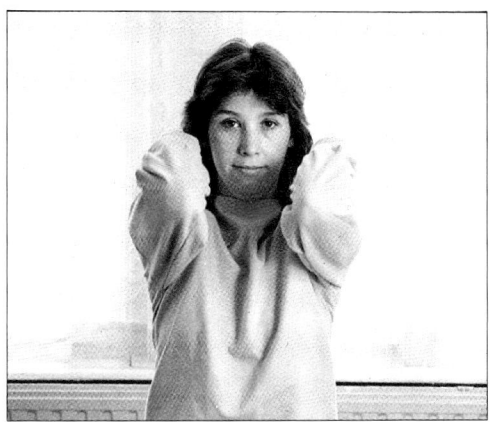
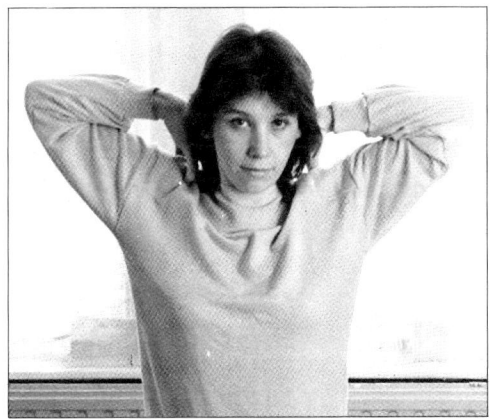
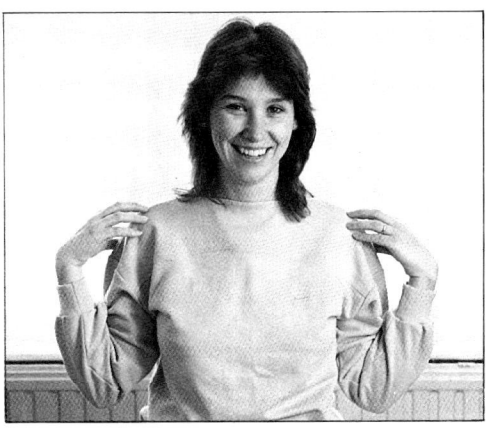
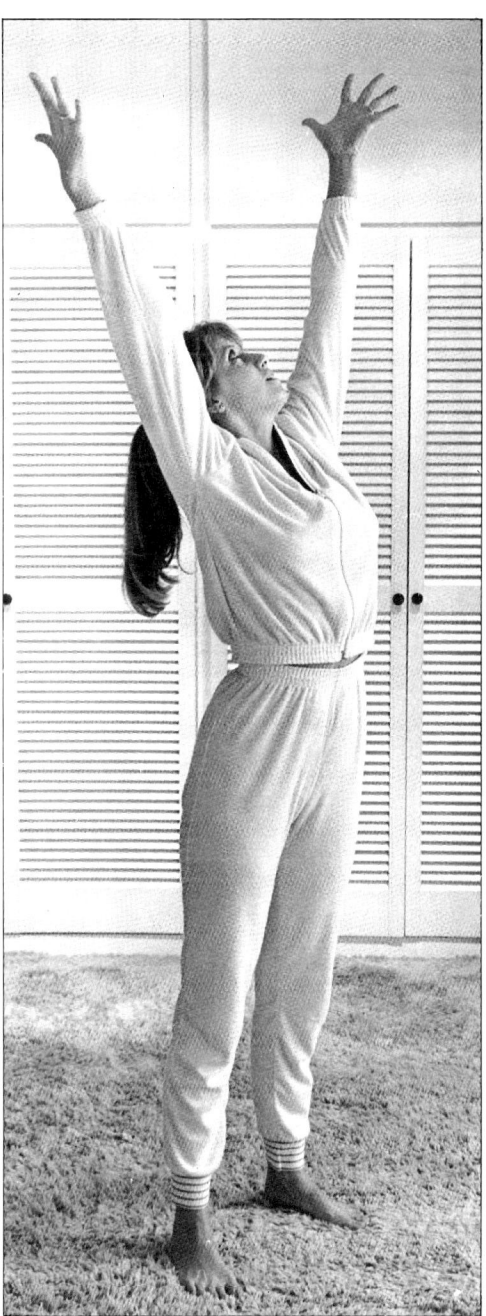

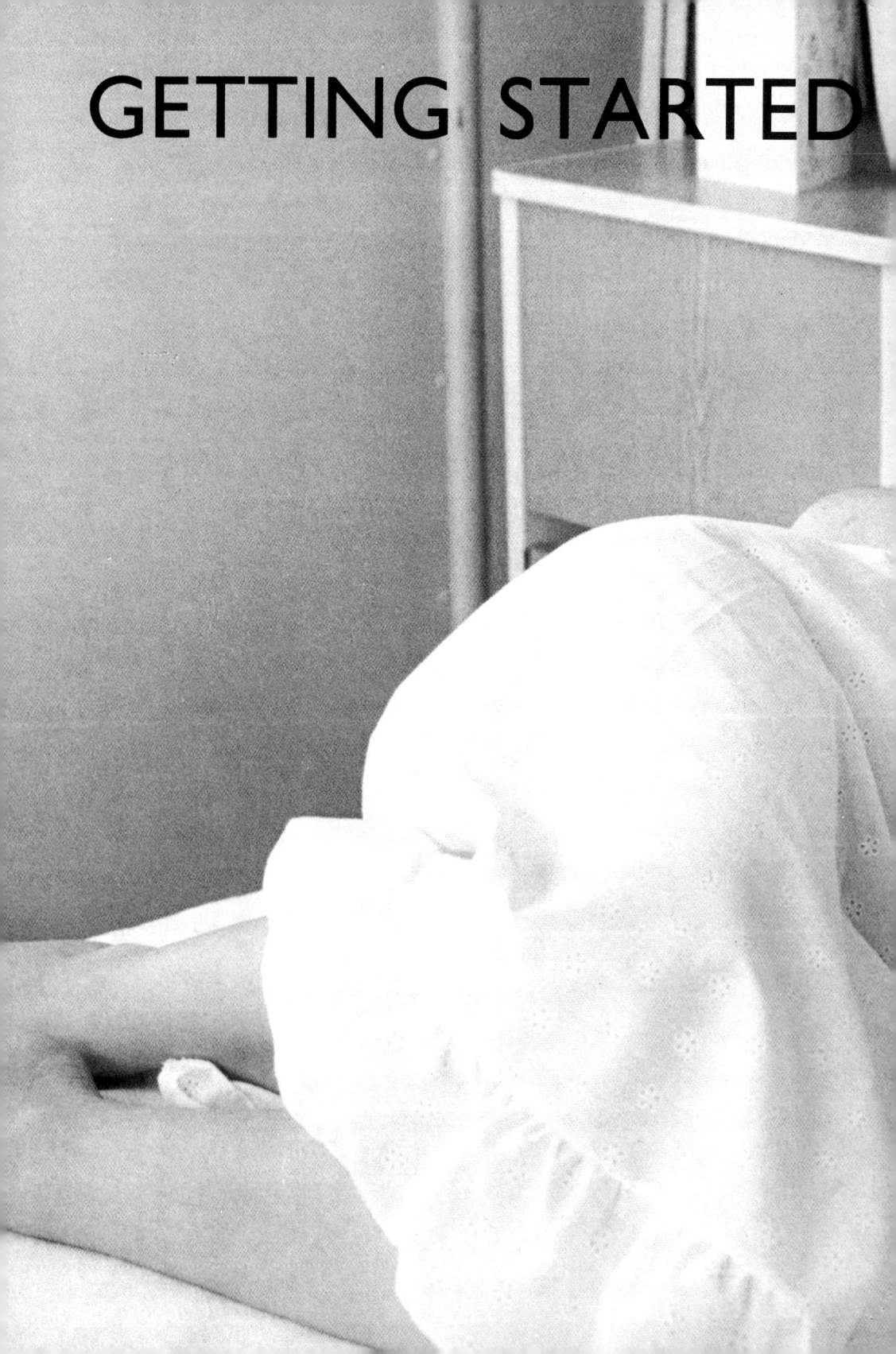

GETTING STARTED

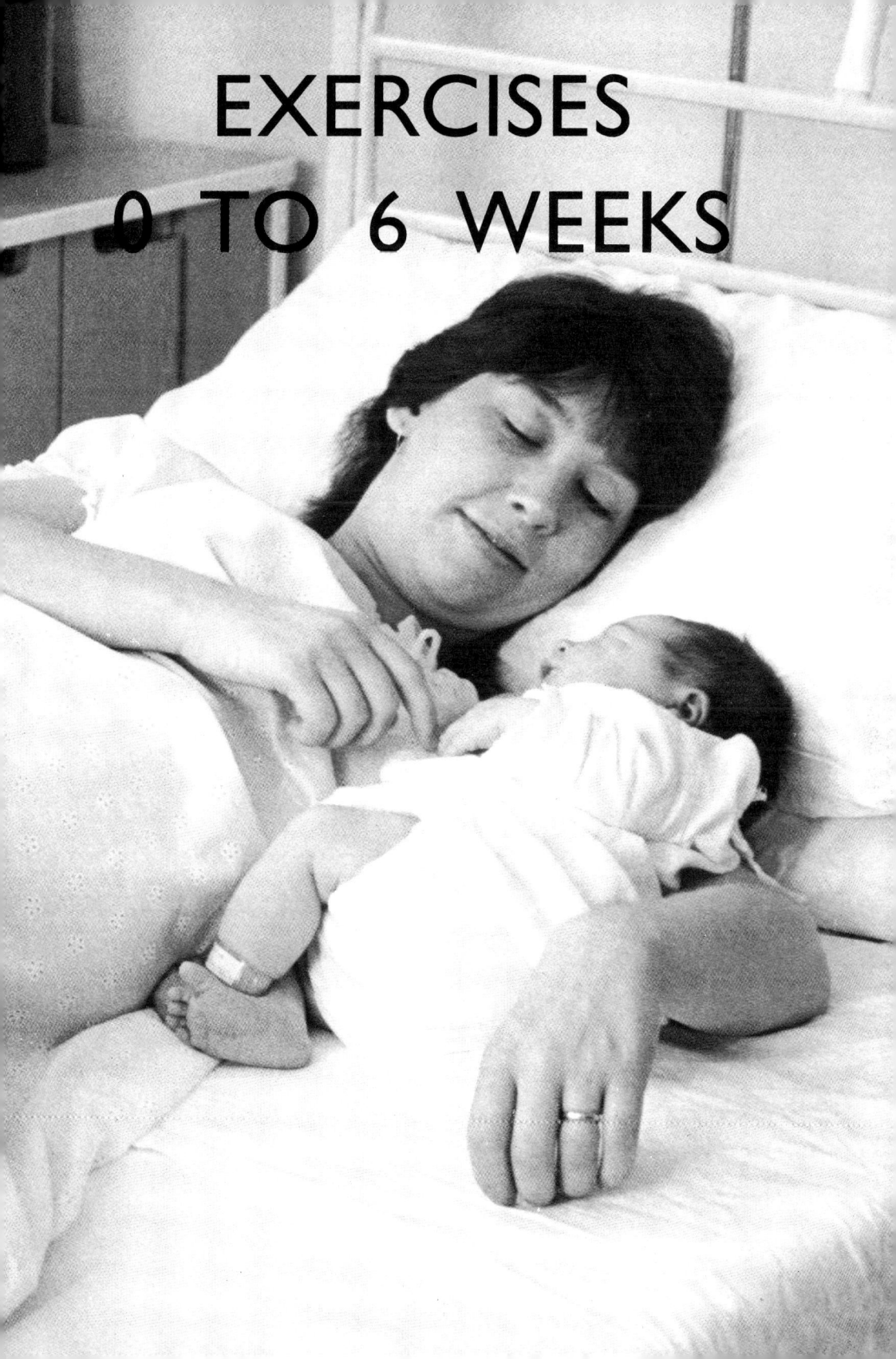

EXERCISES
0 TO 6 WEEKS

First thoughts on exercise

You won't feel like starting a vigorous program of postnatal exercises for quite a while after your baby is born. It is important though to begin some gentle movements at once, whatever sort of delivery you have had, partly to make you more comfortable, but also to begin to strengthen your lengthened, separated abdominal muscles and your weak pelvic floor.

You may have little or no discomfort, or you may experience heavy legs, a sore, throbbing perineum, and, possibly, backache. If you have had a Caesarean section there may be intense burning pain over and around the line of the incision. Whatever your type of delivery, you will probably notice that every time you try to change your position during the first few hours, there will be a flow of blood (lochia) from the vagina. This may make you feel nervous about moving, let alone beginning your exercises. If you have stitches in your pelvic floor or abdomen, you may also be worried that they will come apart if you move too energetically. However, you can be quite sure that all the exercises given in the first part (the first 48 hours) of this section are not only safe but essential for your speedy recovery and you can even do the first four while still in the delivery room.

Exercise while you feed

After the first few days you won't have the time or energy for a regular exercise session, so try and fit in a few exercises when you can. Get into the habit of drawing in your abdominal muscles and pulling your pelvic floor muscles in and up every time you feed your baby. Aim at twenty strong contractions of each in groups of five at a time (see pages 49 and 52). Make sure you continue all the exercises, except the foot exercises, for the first few weeks.

Afterpains

Many new mothers experience painful uterine contractions ("afterpains") for the first few days, particularly while they are breastfeeding. This is due to the release of the hormone oxytocin, which shrinks the uterus as it stimulates the "let down" reflex in the breast. Women who are bottle-feeding may notice these contractions when they begin abdominal exercises. Although uncomfortable, these are normal and beneficial. Use the exercise described on page 49 to "breathe your way through" the pain.

Being careful

Once you are able to exercise more vigorously there are a few important rules to observe:
1 Never exercise to the point of pain or exhaustion.
2 Stop if you feel nauseated, dizzy, or faint.
3 Learn to listen to your body so that you do not inadvertently strain your weak muscles.
4 Don't exercise last thing at night when you are feeling tired, or if you are ill and have a raised temperature.

A warning

There are two exercises that should **never** be attempted during this postnatal period. They are:
1 Lying flat on your back with both legs straight on the floor, and then trying to lift them together.
2 Lying flat on your back with both legs straight and attempting to sit up.

THE FIRST FORTY-EIGHT HOURS

BREATHING AND FIRST ABDOMINAL EXERCISE

This exercise improves your circulation, gently shortens and strengthens your abdominal muscles, and helps you relax.

Lie comfortably on your back with your knees bent, resting your hand on your abdomen. Take a slow, deep breath in through your nose, then sigh the air out through your slightly parted lips and draw your abdominal muscles in at the end of the outward breath. Some women are surprised that these muscles should be pulled in at this point, but it is in fact part of the natural breathing pattern. Once you have learned this sequence, you will then be able to use your outward breath to help you relax.

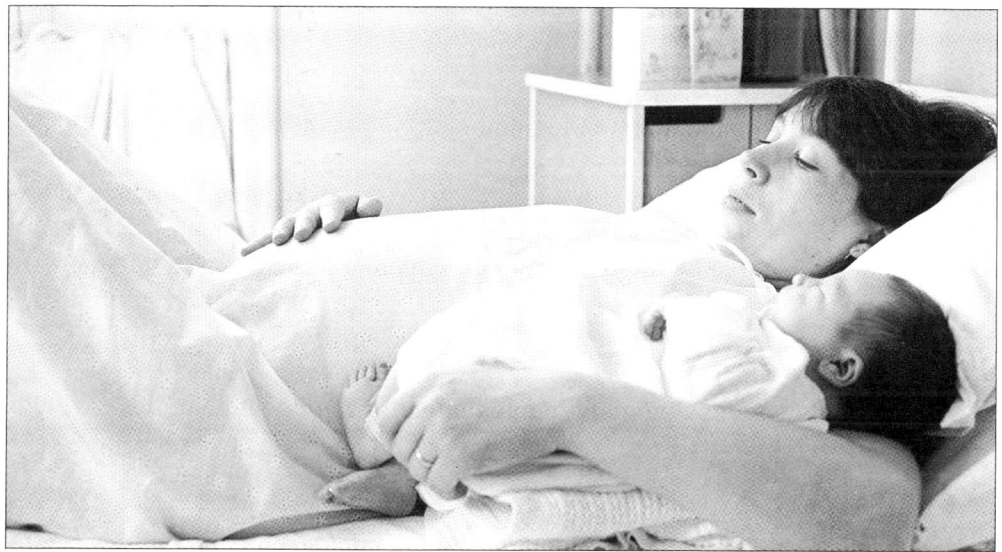

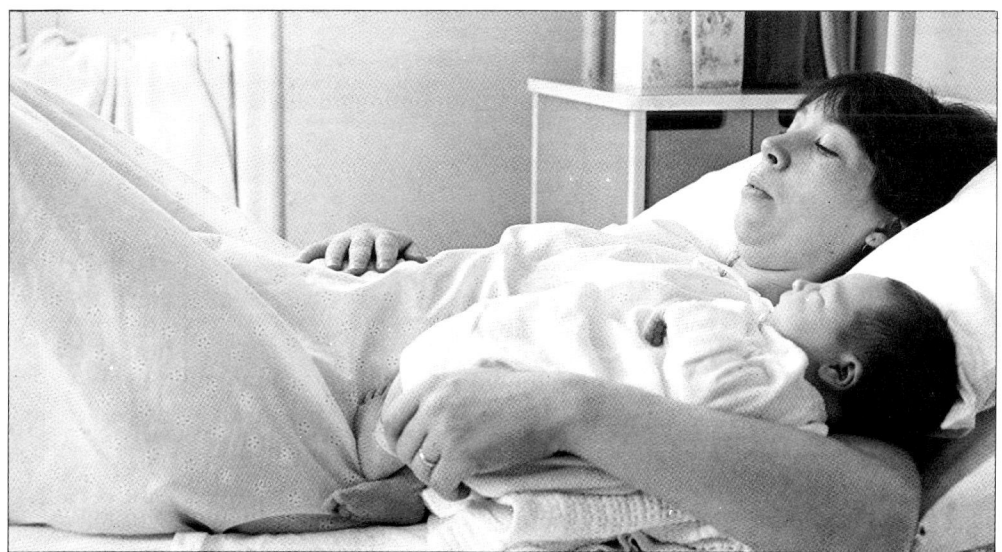

SIDE-LYING CURLS

This is the first step toward shortening and firming your lax abdominal muscles.

Lie on your side with your knees bent. Breathe out and draw your abdominal muscles in, rounding your back; then relax and allow your waist to hollow. Start with six and increase to twenty, roll over and repeat on the other side.

Rhythmically rocking your pelvis back and forth like this can relieve backache too. Progress by holding your abdominal muscles in while you count to five; don't hold your breath, but breathe gently as you draw in. Later, you can try pulling your pelvic floor muscles in and up as you round your back. This is an ideal feeding exercise.

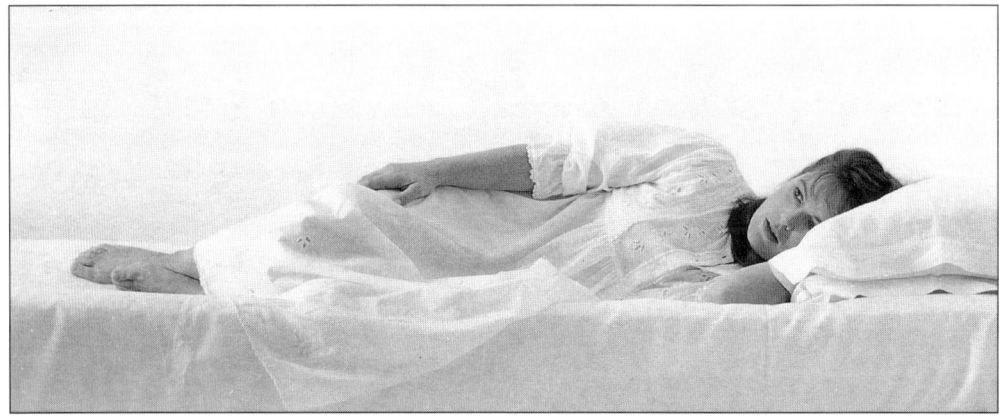

FOOT EXERCISES

These movements will improve your leg circulation; they are particularly important if you have to stay in bed.

Lie comfortably with your knees straight and your feet about 12 in (30 cm) apart. Now bend and stretch your feet up and down at the ankles (right and below right). This should be done briskly and for about thirty seconds at a time. Then circle your feet eight times in each direction (below).

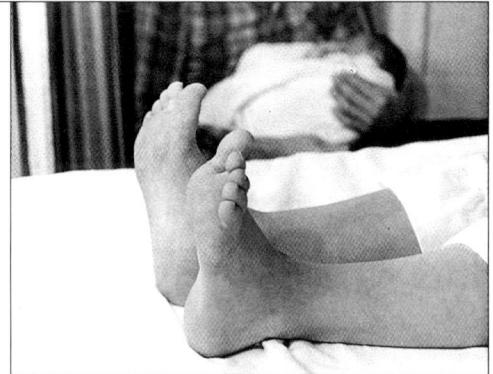

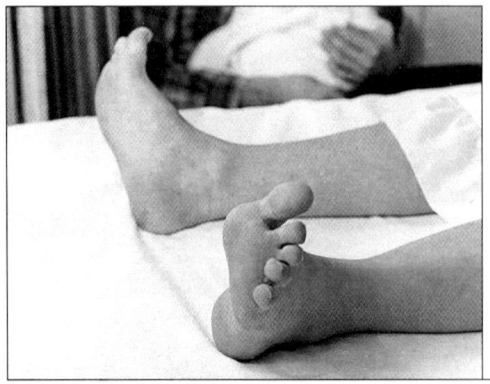

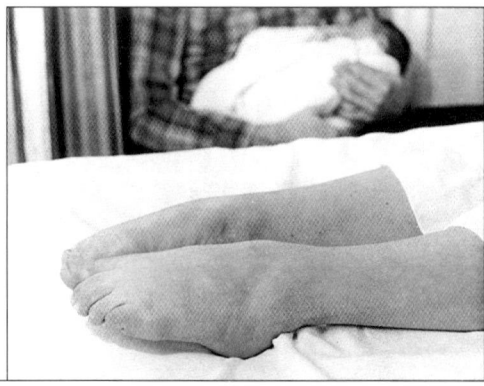

REVERSE PELVIC THRUSTS

This exercise shortens and firms the abdominal muscles. It can help ease backache, constipation, and post-Caesarean section abdominal gas.

Lie comfortably with knees bent and together. Blow out, draw in your abdominal muscles, squeeze your buttock muscles together, tilting your bottom up, and press your back firmly onto the bed. Hold for four counts. When you feel able, this exercise can be made more difficult by holding the muscle contractions for up to ten counts, and lifting your head from the pillow. You can include a pelvic tuck too (page 52).

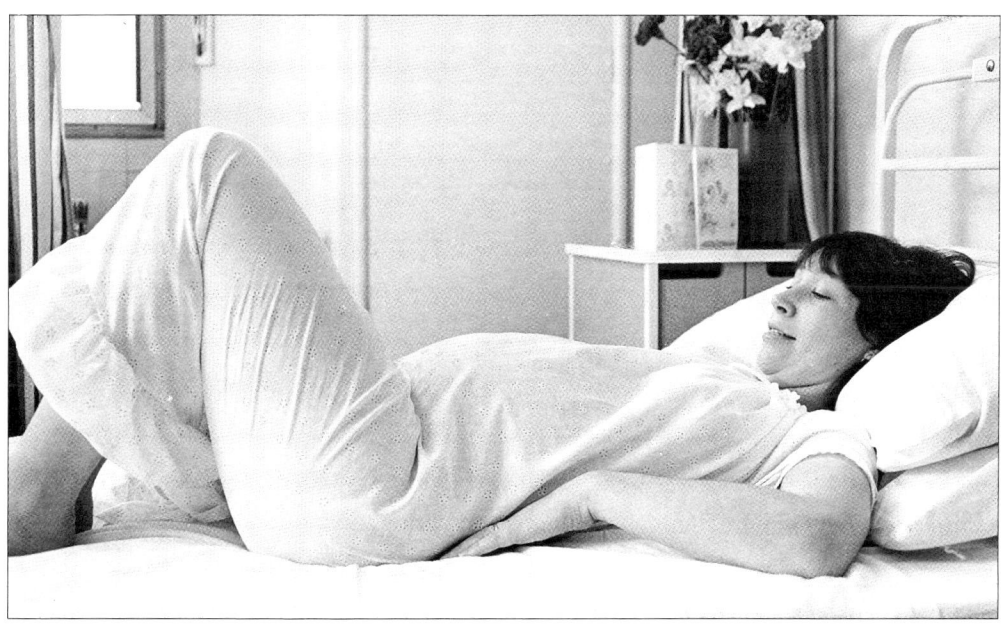

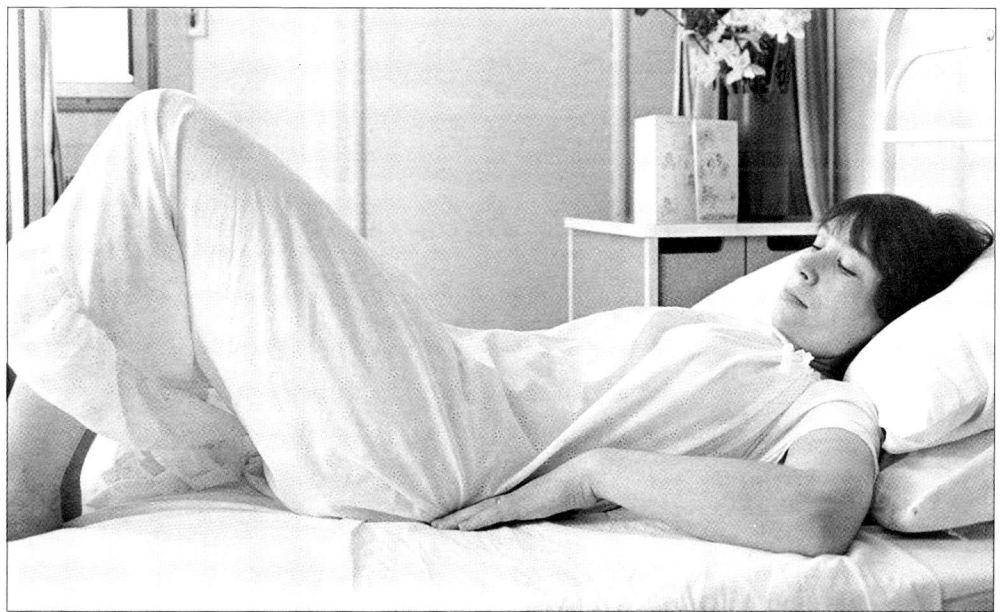

PELVIC TUCKS

This most important exercise strengthens the pelvic floor muscles, and helps relieve pain by improving circulation so that swelling is absorbed.

Lie with your knees bent and apart. At first you may be unable to feel your vagina, so start by squeezing shut your anus as if holding back gas, then let it relax. Next, imagine a tampon is falling out of your vagina. Draw your vaginal muscles in and up as if to grip it and stop your urine flow too. Hold, then relax. Now repeat this quick movement more slowly, holding the muscle contraction for two to three seconds. Try to do these contractions at least four times every fifteen minutes. As your muscles get stronger, hold the squeeze for four to five seconds. In the same way that you have become used to a new body posture – bottom tucked in, ribs well lifted – so you should be aware of your pelvic floor, your *internal* posture.

Test your progress occasionally by trying to slow or stop the flow of urine toward the end of your stream.

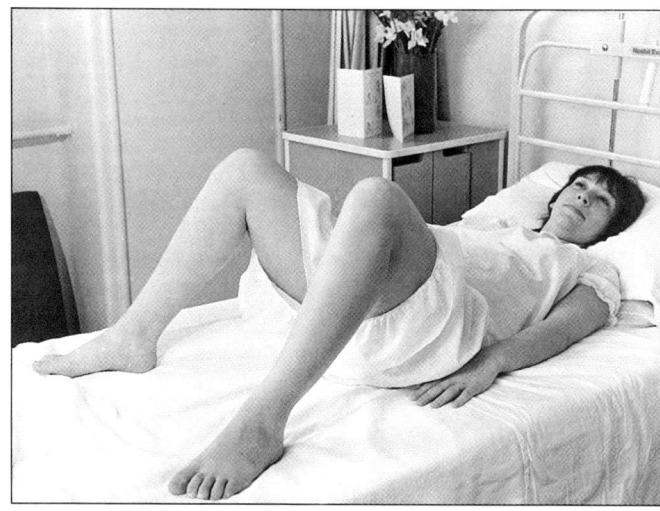

TESTING YOUR ABDOMINAL MUSCLES

If you turn back to page 19 you will see that the two sides of your abdominal "corset" nearly always separate toward the end of your pregnancy to accommodate your growing baby. After your baby's birth this gap can be an indication of the strength of the recti abdominis (the vertical abdominal muscles).

You cannot feel the separation properly unless you make your muscles work hard. To test yourself, lie on your back with your knees bent up high. Put three fingers of one hand just below your umbilicus. Lift your head and shoulders and stretch your other arm toward your feet and feel for the space. Initially almost everyone will have a gap at least three fingers wide – and many women will have a much wider space, four or more fingers wide. Try doing this test once or twice a week. As your muscles recover and become stronger, the gap will gradually close until it is small and tight enough to insert only one or two fingers.

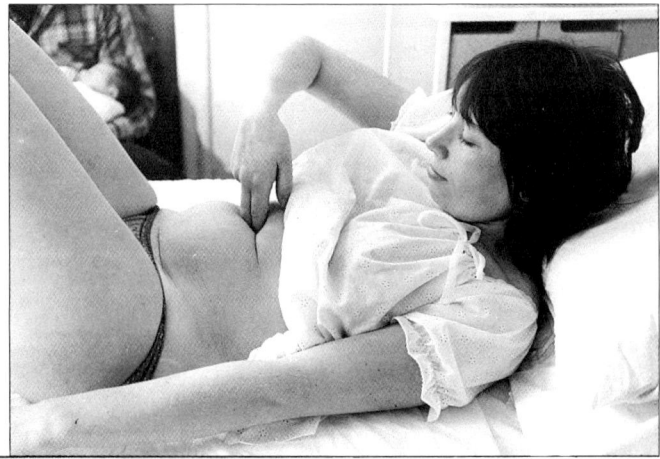

CURL-UPS

This strengthens your recti abdominis muscles (see page 19) and helps close the gap between them.

Lie on your back with knees bent up high. Blow out and tilt your pelvis up by pulling in your abdominal muscles and drawing your buttocks together. Tuck your chin on your chest, and lift your head and shoulders, stretching your hands toward your feet. Hold this position for four counts – and then lower slowly. Start with six and increase to twenty.

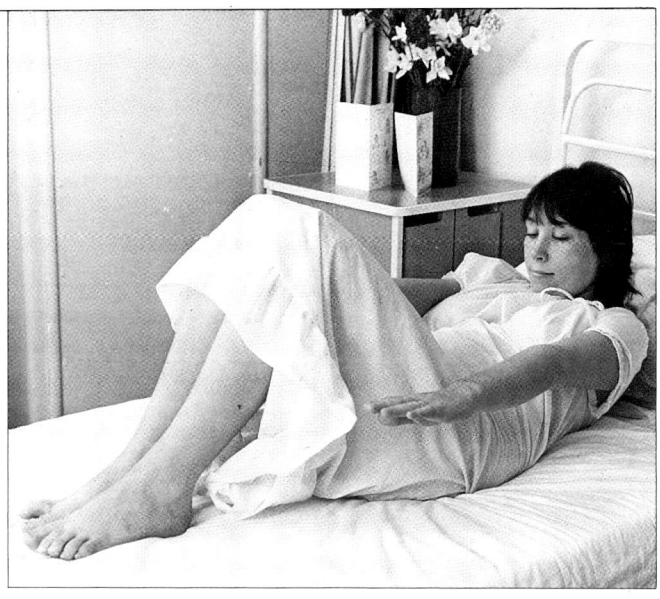

USEFUL RESTING POSITION AND BUTTOCK TUCKS

Many women do not realize that once again they can lie flat on their fronts. To do this really comfortably you will need to use two pillows – one under your waist and the other under your head and shoulders, making a space for your breasts. Of course, this position does not flatten or strengthen your abdomen in any way, but it is very comfortable. Try it for fifteen to thirty minutes every day. If you have a tender episiotomy, hemorrhoids, or backache, you will find that rhythmical buttock-squeezing while lying on your front may help relieve your discomfort. Everyone will eventually find this a restful position, even those who have had a Caesarean section. It will allow you to relax fully without uncomfortable pressure and could begin toning up flabby buttocks.

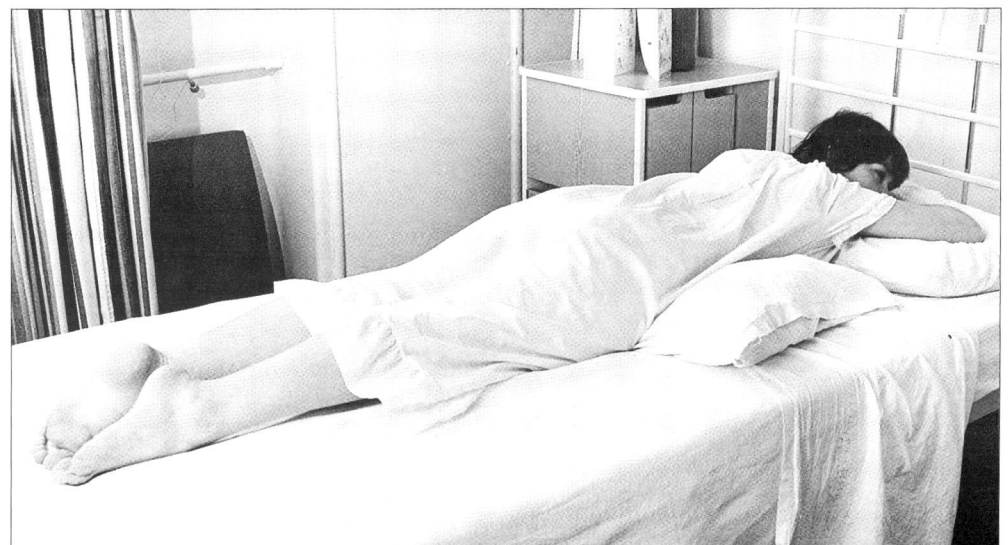

THE POST-CAESAREAN MOTHER

There are two kinds of Caesarean birth:

Elective – you knew in advance that you would have to have a Caesarean section for your baby to be born safely.

Emergency – the decision to help your baby out by Caesarean section was only made during labor.

You may have had a general anesthetic for the operation and could be a bit congested afterward because of its effect on your lungs. Alternatively, you may have had an epidural anesthetic and will have been awake as your baby was born. No matter why or how you had a Caesarean section, you will feel very sore around the site of the operation and will find it very difficult to move easily because of the pain. You will need much more help during the first few days, so ask for it.

Special post-operative exercises

You will feel much better if you do these simple exercises as soon as possible. They will improve your circulation and are relaxing. Lie comfortably on your back, well supported by pillows, with your legs straight.

1 Bend and stretch your ankles vigorously thirty times.
2 Circle your ankles (ten times in each direction).
3 Press your knees down hard and relax (ten times).
4 Draw your buttocks tightly together and relax (ten times).
5 Bend and stretch your knees alternately (ten times).
6 Practice deep breathing, filling and emptying both lungs completely. Try a "huffing" breath outward, while supporting your incision with both hands, if you need to clear your throat.
7 If you are congested, you will need to cough properly. Probably the most comfortable position for coughing is sitting with your legs over the side of your bed or on a high chair. Separate your knees, support your wound with a pillow, *lean forward*, and cough with a sharp "huff."

A pillow placed under your thighs will prevent you from slipping down the bed and another resting across your wound will help prevent too much pain as you feed your baby, or you may like to tuck your baby under your arm with his feet behind you, as shown.

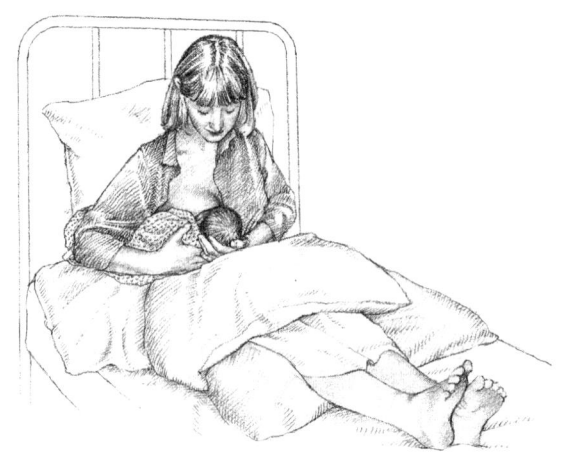

Hints for comfort

Getting in and out of bed

For the first few days you will be most comfortable in bed, well propped up with pillows, or sitting in an armchair.

Make sure that your bed is as low as possible or use a stool. To get out of bed from a reclining position, use your hands and feet to push, not pull, yourself upright. Shuffle your bottom to the edge of the bed and lift your legs one at a time over the side (using your hands if needed). Separate your knees, support your wound with your hands, lean forward and slowly stand up. The first few times you will need some help. After a few days you will be able to lie flat. Then it is easiest to roll on your side to get out of bed – bend your knees and use your arms to push yourself up before swinging your legs over the edge and standing up.

To get back into bed, lower yourself onto the mattress *right next to your pillows*. Make sure your bottom is well on the bed and not on the edge. Now lift your legs one at a time onto the bed, using your hands if necessary.

Standing and walking

You will probably have to support your wound with your hands in the beginning – but if you can straighten up it is usually less painful. Practice deep, slow breathing as you move around the room and go to the bathroom.

Feeding your baby

Sit up in bed, or on a chair, well supported by pillows. Resting a pillow across your abdomen protects your wound from the weight of your baby. Like many post-Caesarean mothers, you may be more comfortable with your baby tucked under your arm.

Pain

After your Caesarean section you will probably have pain from at least three sources: your wound, "afterpains" (see page 48), and abdominal gas.

Solutions

1 You should be offered mild painkillers. Don't reject these – there is no virtue in suffering and they won't affect your baby.
2 To relieve gas, stroke your abdomen from the right groin up to just below your ribs, across your abdomen to your left side and down to your left groin. Repeat this, gently pushing the gas along your large bowel, until you can pass it.
3 Reverse pelvic thrusts (see page 51) will also ease gas discomfort.
4 Roll your knees gently from side to side (see page 77).

Normal postnatal exercising

Your doctor will guide you. You will probably only be a little behind the other mothers, but because you have had a major operation as well as having had a baby it will take you longer to recover from the birth than your friends who have had vaginal deliveries. It is important to accept that you will need to take things easy for the first four weeks or longer.

At home

When you first go home, rest as much as possible and try to make the household chores wait until you feel better. If family and friends offer to shop, clean, or cook for you, or take your other children off your hands for a while, do accept their help.

As the weeks go by you will find that you gradually feel stronger and more able to cope – you will have caught up with mothers whose babies were born through the vagina.

AFTER TWO TO THREE DAYS

SITTING PELVIC ROCKS

This shortens your vertical abdominal muscles, helps to close the gap between them, and relieves backache.

Sit on the edge of a chair with your legs apart, resting your hands on your knees. Breathe out and draw your abdominal muscles in as hard as you can, rounding your back into a banana shape; relax and allow your spine to hollow gently. Repeat six times and increase to twenty. Progress by holding in for five to ten seconds, breathing gently as you do so.

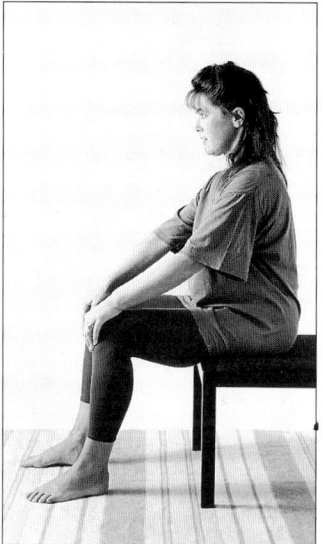 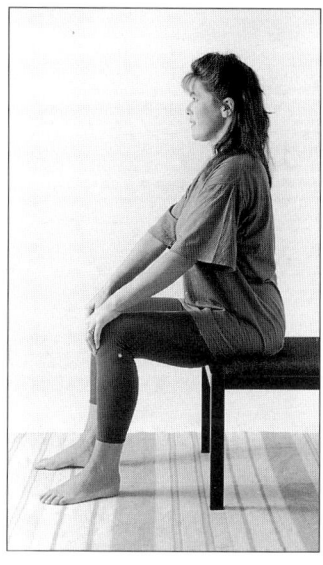

LATERAL BENDS

This exercise works the muscles at the sides and front of your waist.

Sit up straight on a chair with your knees and feet apart. Hold your abdomen in firmly and keep your bottom fixed on the chair. Bend sideways to the right without allowing your body to lean forward or back. Stretch your hand toward the floor. Keeping your stomach flat, straighten up slowly, then relax your abdomen. Repeat the movement to the left. Do this four times to each side, increasing to twenty.

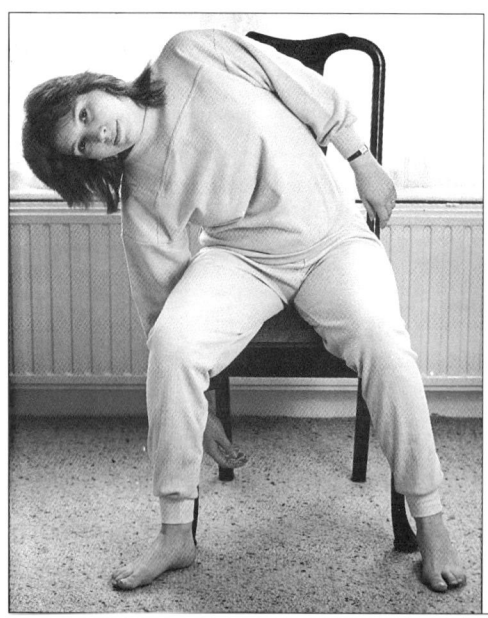 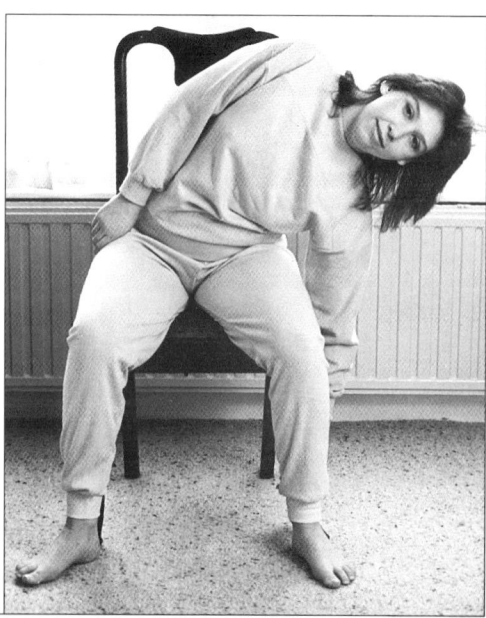

WAIST TWISTERS

This exercise uses the diagonal (oblique) abdominal muscles; it helps to pull in your waist and mobilize your spine.

Sit up straight on a chair with your knees and feet apart and your arms lifted and bent in front of you. With your bottom fixed on the chair and your back erect, pull your abdomen in hard. Now, twist to the right as far as you can; count to four, then twist to the left; count to four; return to the middle and relax your abdominal muscles. Do this six times to each side, increasing to twenty.

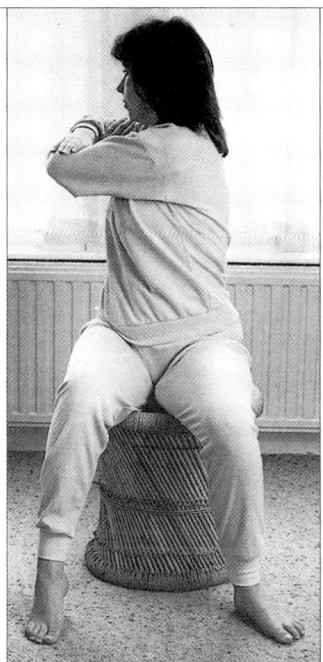 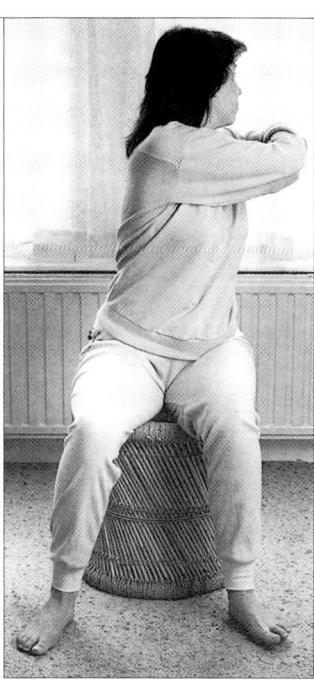

ALTERNATE KNEE LIFTS

This exercise will help shorten and firm your vertical abdominal muscles (recti abdominis).

Sit on the edge of a chair, resting your hands lightly on the back of the seat, and bend your elbows. Draw your abdominal muscles in firmly; round your spine, lean back a little, and raise your right knee.

Now change legs so that your left leg comes up as your right leg goes down – breathe easily throughout the exercise.

Start with ten and increase to twenty. To make it harder, as your abdominal muscles get stronger, lift your arms in front of you clasping your hands together. Do twenty leg changes, pause, do another twenty.

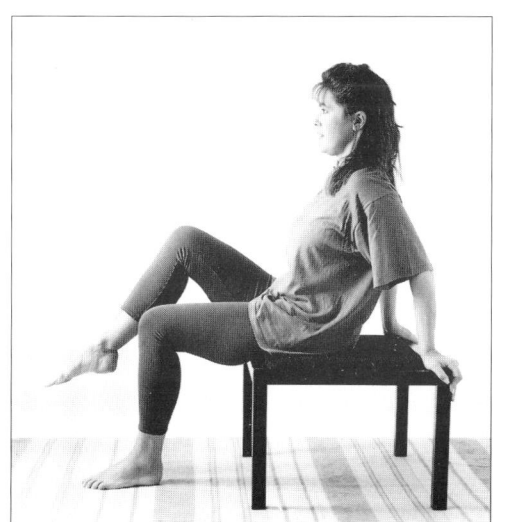 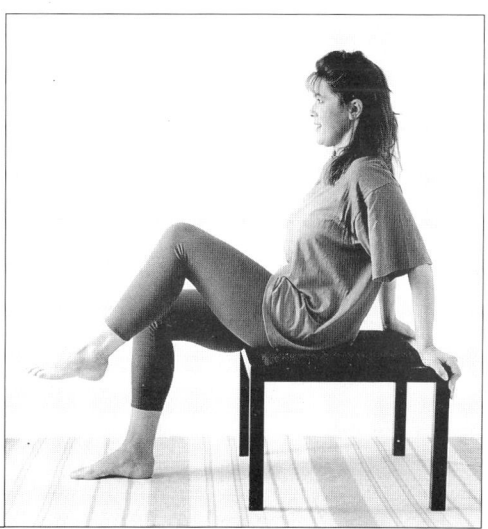

PECTORAL TONERS

When you first do this exercise it will probably be helpful to watch yourself in a mirror. You should see a brisk movement of the muscles underlying the breasts, and some women may notice them move too.

Sit in the same position as for the Waist Twisters (see page 57). Push the palms of your hands firmly against your upper arms and stop. You will feel your pectoral (chest) muscles contracting and then relaxing. Do this ten times to start with, increasing to twenty.

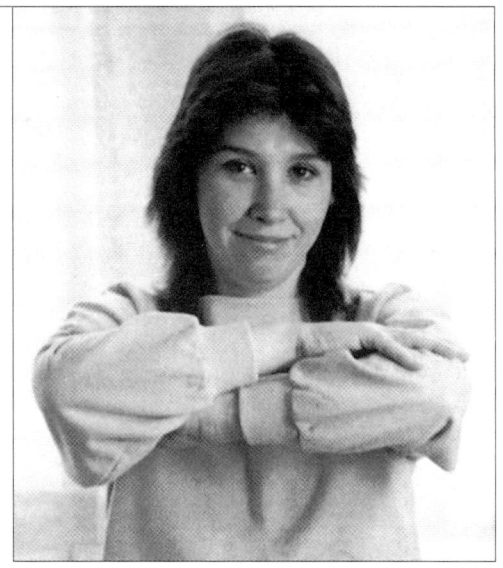

SEATED BACK EXTENSIONS

This useful exercise can be done almost anywhere and at any time to achieve quick relaxation. It has the added benefit of loosening your tired, tense back muscles.

Sit straight on a chair or stool with your knees and feet wide apart. Curl forward, breathing out, so that your arms and head are hanging heavily down. Relax in this position for a few moments, breathing quietly, feeling the tension draining out of you. Then slowly uncurl your body, straightening your lower back and waist first, followed by your shoulders and finally your head. Hold this relaxed but upright position for a moment, making sure that your shoulders are not hunched up by your ears.

Repeat this slow curling and uncurling movement a few times until your back feels comfortable and easy.

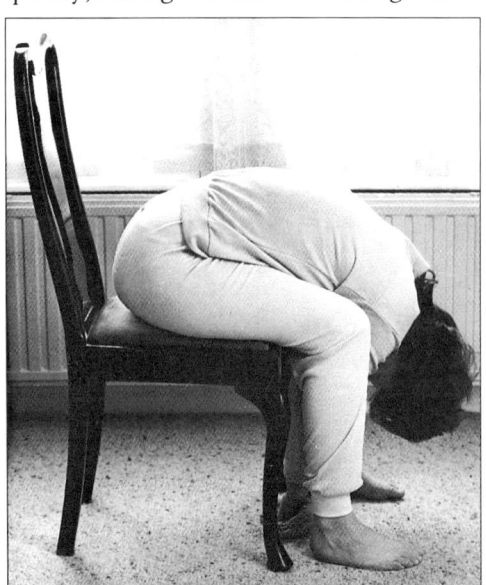
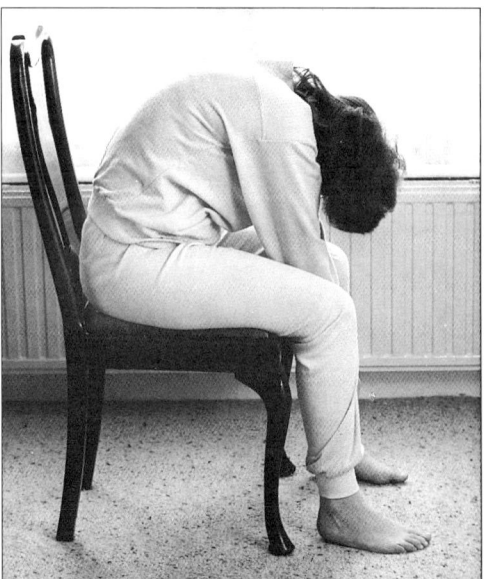

STANDING PELVIC ROCKS

This exercise shortens and strengthens your vertical abdominal muscles and eases backache.

Stand with your feet apart, bend your knees, and rest your hands lightly on your thighs. Breathe out, draw your abdominal muscles in hard and round your back. Relax and arch your spine behind your waist. Repeat rhythmically, breathing out as you draw your abdomen in and breathing in as you arch. Start with six, and increase to twenty. Progress by holding in your abdomen for five seconds, breathing easily as you do so.

To correct your posture, straighten your knees, lift your ribs, draw your abdomen in, and tuck your bottom under.

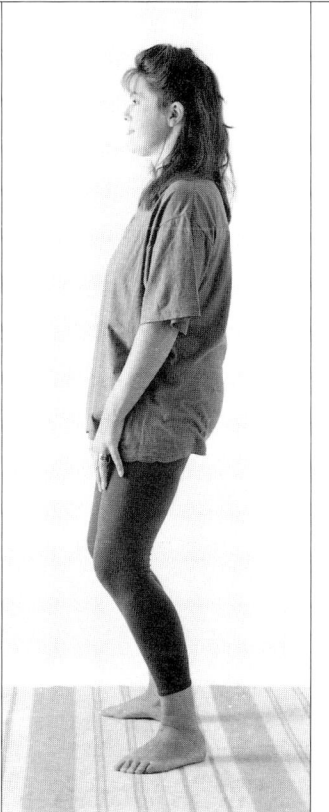
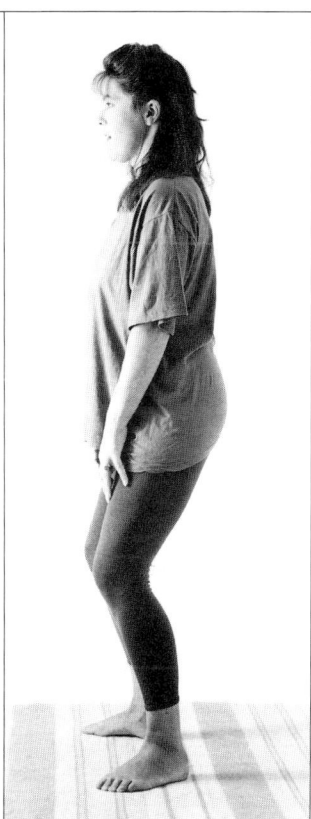

HIP-CIRCLING

Circling your hips uses all your abdominal muscles and makes your lower back muscles work too. As well as helping to shorten and strengthen stretched, weakened muscles, this exercise mobilizes your lower spine and can relieve a tired, aching lower back.

Stand with your feet about 12 in (30 cm) apart, bend your knees a little, and rest your hands on your hips.

Now circle your hips to the right, forward, to the left, round to the back, and then to the right again. Take your pelvis all the way around in a big, slow, controlled circle. As your hips come forward draw your abdomen in really hard, making your straight abdominal muscles work extra strongly. Do ten circles to the right and then ten slow, large circles to the left. Progress to twenty in each direction.

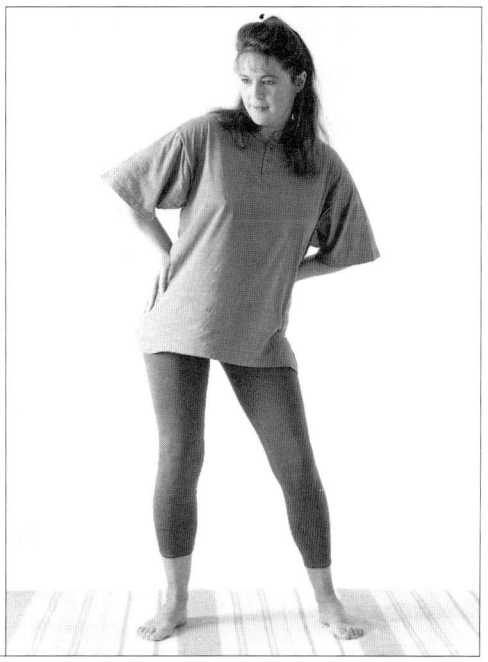

SUPINE LEG SLIDES

This exercise strengthens and firms your vertical abdominal muscles and helps close the gap between them.

Lie on the floor with your fingers behind your head, your palms over your ears. Bend your left knee up high. Breathe out, drawing your abdominal muscles in firmly and raise your head, tucking your chin onto your chest. Now change legs so that your left slides down as your right comes up; then lower your head.

Start with one leg change for each head lift and repeat ten times. Progress by changing your legs twice, then four, six, eight, or ten times for each head raise; later, lift your legs instead of sliding them. Breathe easily as you exercise.

Try alternate leg-sliding in the bath!

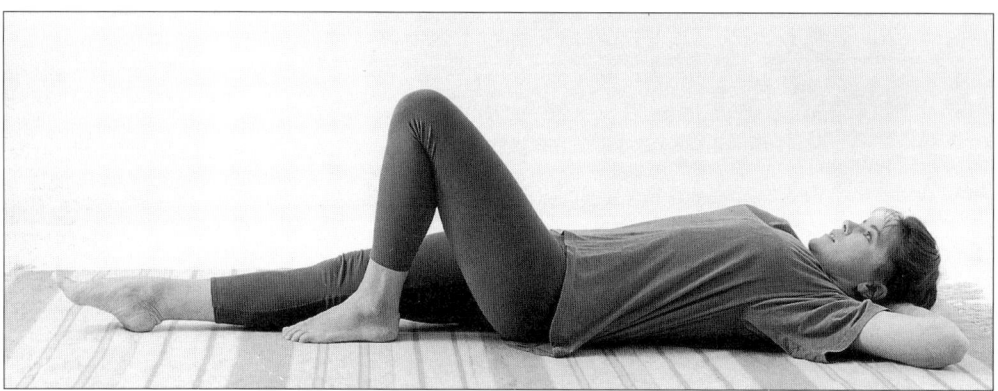

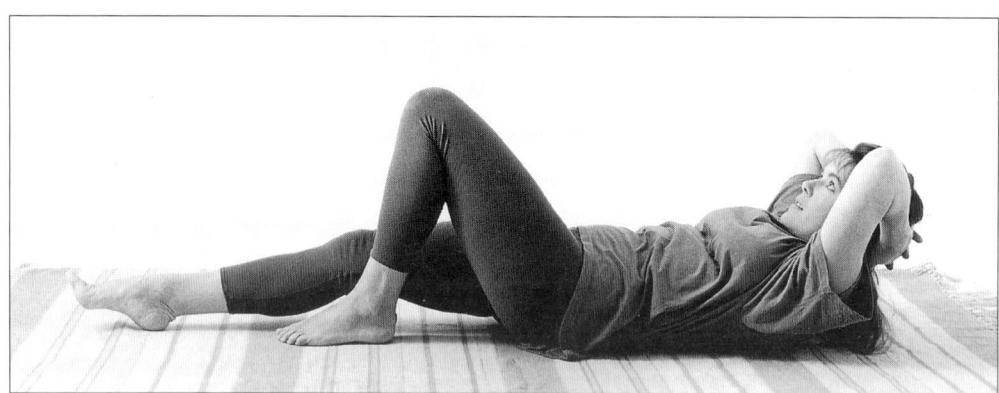

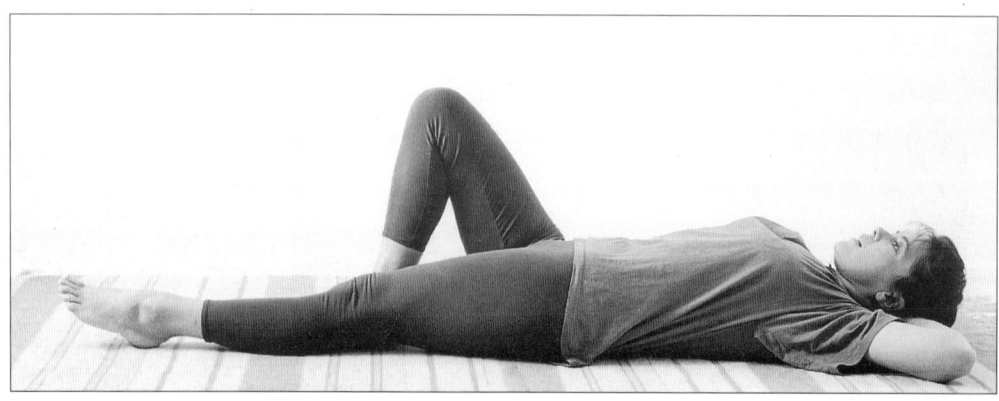

PRONE LEG HYPEREXTENSIONS

This exercise helps firm your buttocks, strengthens the important muscles of your lower back, improves your posture, and helps relieve backache.

Lie flat on your front on the floor with your head resting on your hands. If your breasts are full and tender, relieve pressure and make a space for them by putting a pillow under your head and shoulders and another under your ribs. Keeping your knee straight, lift your left leg without allowing your pelvis to twist sideways. Hold for four counts and lower. Now do the same with your right leg.

Lift each leg alternately, ten times, increasing to twenty. If you experience back pain while doing this exercise, try putting an extra pillow under your waist.

You can make this exercise harder by lowering the working leg to about 6 in (15 cm) or so from the floor and then lifting it again; work faster and do twenty on each leg.

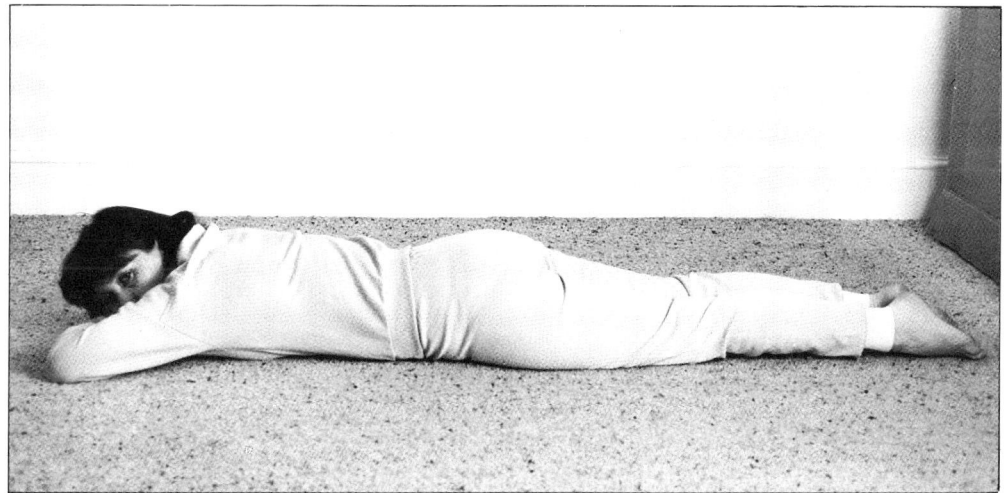

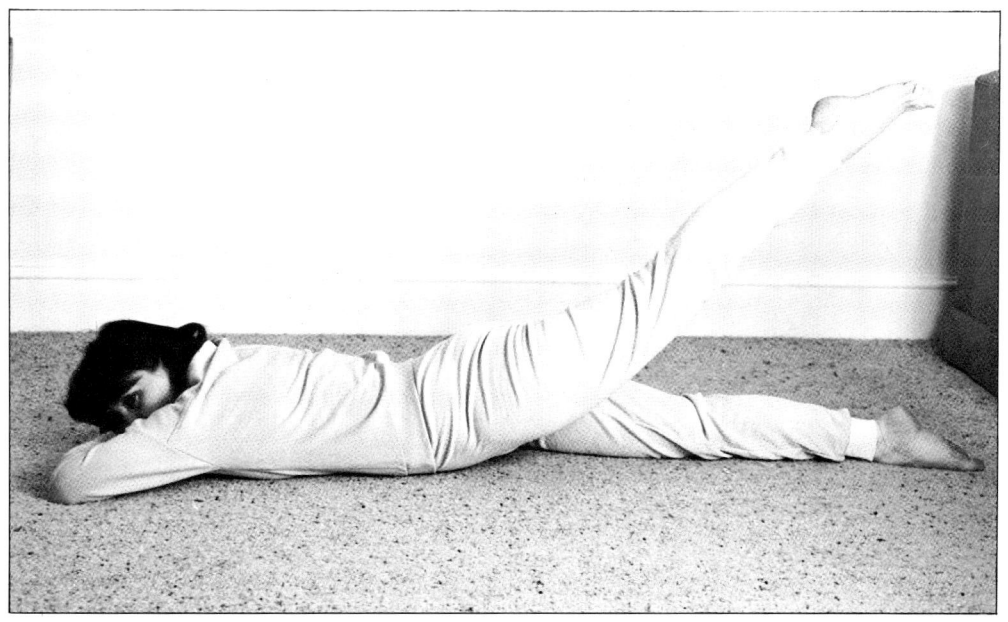

DAILY PROGRAM

We suggest you do the following exercises two or three times a day unless otherwise stated. Asterisks mark the most important ones. Initially, post-Caesarean section mothers should also do the exercises on page 54.

The first 48 hours

BREATHING AND FIRST ABDOMINAL EXERCISE
Circulation, abdominal muscles, relaxation page 49
Do this 4 times every so often

*SIDE-LYING CURLS
Abdominal muscles, backache page 50
6 to 20 on each side; continue doing this exercise for several weeks

FOOT EXERCISES
Leg circulation page 50
Do the first exercise for 30 seconds, and the second exercise 8 times in each direction, 3 to 4 times a day; discontinue after 2 days, unless your ankles are swollen

*REVERSE PELVIC THRUSTS
Abdominal and buttock muscles page 51
10 to 20 rocks

*PELVIC TUCKS
Pelvic floor muscles page 52
Throughout the day

TESTING YOUR ABDOMINAL MUSCLES
page 52
Try doing this test once or twice a week and note the gradual change

*CURL-UPS
Vertical abdominal muscles page 53
10 to 20 times

RESTING POSITION AND BUTTOCK TUCKS
Buttocks, backache page 53
Use the resting position for 15 to 30 minutes; squeeze your buttocks 10 times every so often while you rest

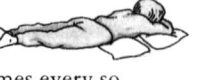

After 2 to 3 days add:

*SITTING PELVIC ROCKS
Vertical abdominal muscles, backache page 56
Start with 6, increase to 20

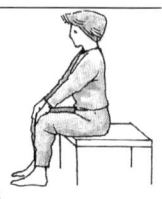

LATERAL BENDS
Side and front waist muscles page 56
4 to 20 each side

WAIST TWISTERS
Oblique abdominal muscles page 57
6 to 20 each side

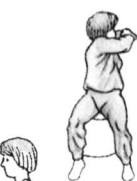

*ALTERNATE KNEE LIFTS
Vertical abdominal muscles page 57 Start with 10, increase to 20

PECTORAL TONERS
Pectoral muscles page 58
10 times, increase to 20

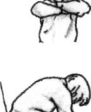

SEATED BACK EXTENSIONS
Relaxation and back muscles page 58
Repeat a few times

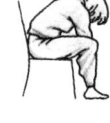

*STANDING PELVIC ROCKS
Vertical abdominal muscles, backache page 59
Start with 6, increase to 20

HIP-CIRCLING
Abdominal and lower back muscles, backache page 59
Start with 10 to each side, increase to 20

*SUPINE LEG SLIDES
Vertical abdominal muscles page 60
Start with 10, increase to 20

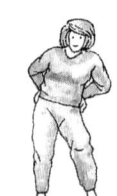
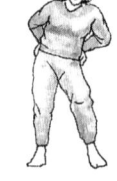

PRONE LEG HYPEREXTENSIONS
Buttocks and lower back muscles page 61
Start with 10, increase to 20 for each leg

Post workout relaxation
Lean on a table to rest (page 42), then practice physiological relaxation (pages 40–41).

YOUR BABY'S EARLY NEEDS

Having left the enfolding security of the womb for the strange, noisy, and vast space of the outside world, your baby will need your warmth and reassurance to help adjust to her new environment. Sudden careless movements will startle her and cause her to throw out her arms involuntarily in panic. Babies like calm, confident handling; being wrapped and held securely nearly always soothes and relaxes them. Swaddling is a time-honored method of making a very new baby feel calm, warm, and contented.

Points to consider In the first six weeks, babies' material needs are few – food, warmth, and clothing, and somewhere comfortable to sleep. It is worthwhile remembering this, for you will probably feel pressured to buy when you walk into a baby store and see all the paraphernalia that manufacturers seem to believe essential for your child's normal development.

You will probably already have some ideas as to the choice of bed and transport for your baby, based on considerations such as whether you have a car, are going back to work and will be leaving your baby with others, have older children, like to stay at home, like to walk everywhere, are glad to make do with hand-me-downs, or want to have only the newest and best that you can afford.

You may have taken advice on the safest and best-designed equipment and toys, but there are some important points to consider from your own physical point of view and also for the development of your baby, which you will not be able to learn from the catalogs.

Keeping your baby amused It is now recognized that full-term newborn babies can see and follow movement with their eyes; they can hear, taste, and smell, and within a matter of days have learned to identify the face, voice, and smell of their mothers. They are, however, completely dependent, and it is only by crying that they are able to convey their needs. Their movements are jerky, uncontrolled, and often governed by infant reflexes. They are passive observers, learning through their senses about the world around them.

By about three or four weeks of age they start to watch their mothers and fathers intently, following them with their eyes, and their own face becomes increasingly alert. They are interested in movement, particularly that of a face, and turn their head toward light, and sometimes to a nearby sound, such as music or a voice. Their body and limbs still remain generally curled up and their hands can only open involuntarily. But by the time they are six weeks old they will enjoy searching their mothers' and fathers' faces – especially their eyes and mouths – and will often hold their gaze for several moments, perhaps even breaking into a lopsided smile.

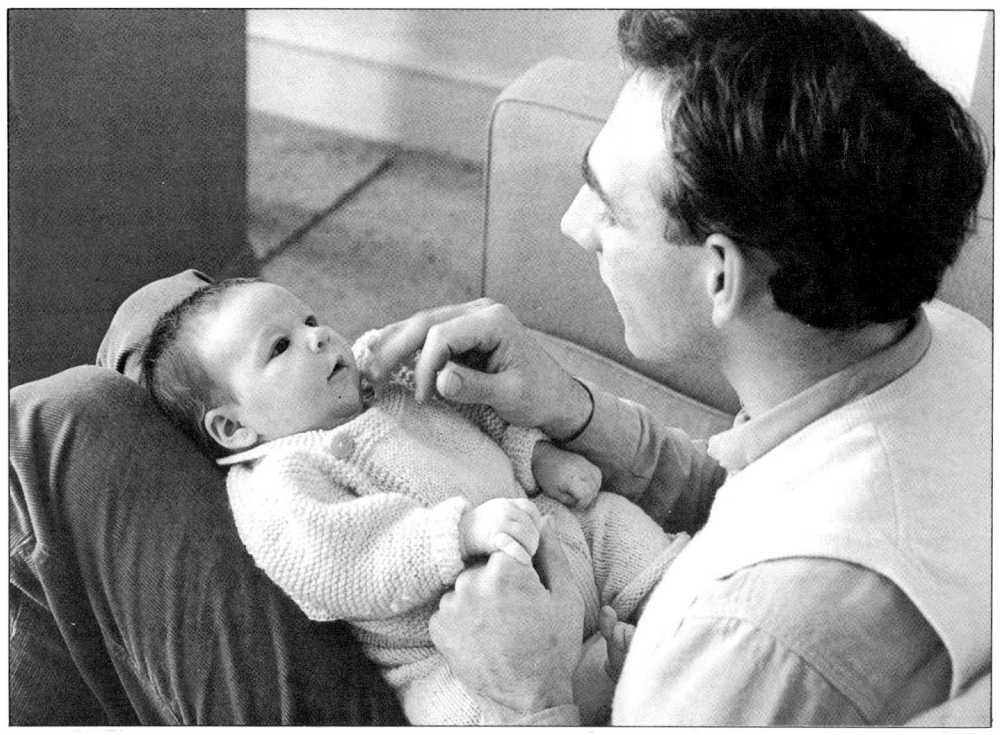

Looking and listening

At this stage babies do not need many toys to play with – they are totally absorbed in learning about their environment, especially the people most important to them. Of course you can't always be available to them if they lie awake, so you can try taping some colorful pictures to the side of the crib or a picture on the wall nearest where they spend most of the day. A mobile, balloons, or a soft toy suspended securely 8–15 in (20–40 cm) above the crib may provide movement and color to catch their interest and help develop sensory awareness, and a rattle can be interesting to listen to, although they won't be able to hold it yet. A music box playing a soothing tune helps to settle some babies. Remember, however, that you are by far the most exciting thing in your baby's world.

Carrying your baby

Baby carriers (or slings) are a comforting and natural way to carry babies. They enjoy the warmth of your body, the reassuring sound of your heartbeat and the motion. Being carried in this way is also physically good for them, as it encourages head control and a healthy position of the hips. Carriers are often an answer for the unsettled or colicky baby, who may cease crying and even fall asleep while her mother manages a few chores. Your partner, and your baby's grandparents and friends, will enjoy using the baby carrier too.

Occasionally, babies do not enjoy baby carriers and protest when put in them, while others do not like long spells in one and demand to be taken out. It is worth trying your baby in the carrier of your choice before buying – some stores encourage this.

Choosing a baby carrier

Be sure when you buy or borrow a baby carrier that it has shoulder straps that are wide, well padded, and adjustable. Position your baby as high as possible on your chest (so you can kiss the top of the baby's head), thus minimizing the strain to your back. The best-designed carriers can be used for a newborn baby (these are worn on the front and offer head support) while adapting to suit a toddler (worn on the back). It is unwise for a new mother, whose back may be especially vulnerable for five to six months, to wear a baby carrier on the side. She should also be prepared to discard it if it gives her low back pain after use.

Carrying with one arm

There is an excellent way of carrying your baby without a baby carrier, but that still leaves one arm free. Using your preferred hand, place your forearm down the front of your baby's trunk with the head resting into the crook of your elbow. The baby's underside arm must be behind your forearm for safety, and your hand can then hold the baby between the legs. This position (see below) stimulates your baby's head control and vision, and you may also find it good for bringing up a burp.

As babies need to experience different ways of lying and being carried, do not keep your baby in one position for too long.

Top left: A baby has begun to focus by six to eight weeks. Remember that your face is your baby's most exciting plaything at this age.

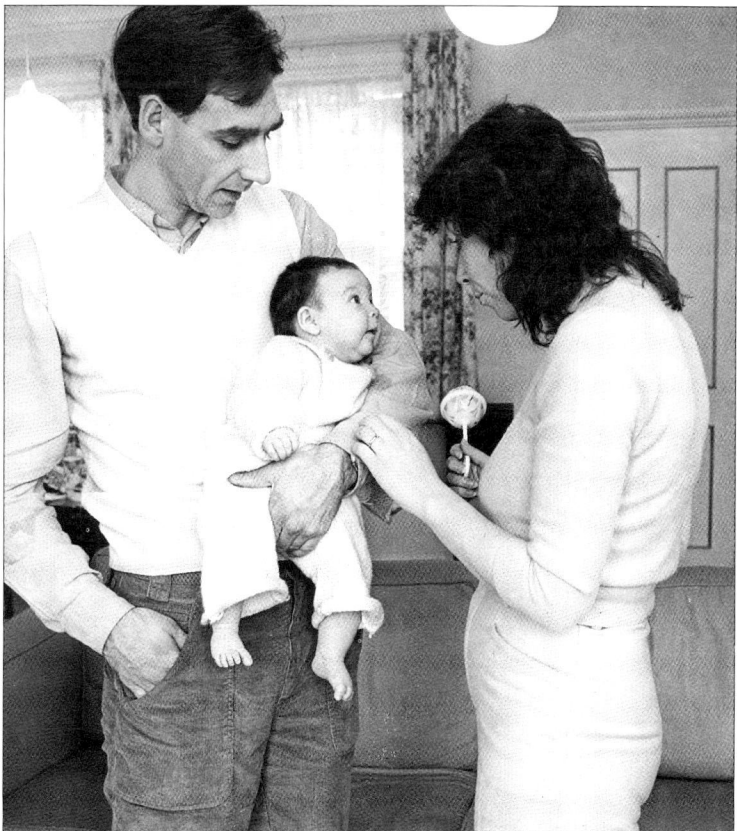

Try this secure way of holding your small baby. It will leave you with a free hand while allowing your baby to watch her surroundings as you move about.

A crying baby

While all babies, particularly very young ones, may swallow air as they feed (especially if they are bottle-fed), and certainly swallow air if they are left to cry, gas is unlikely to be the cause of any incessant crying. Much more likely reasons are hunger, a dirty diaper, feelings of loneliness or over-stimulation, feeling hot or cold, fear of loud noises or being dropped, dislike of being undressed, the urge to suck, and the need to feel a warm body close to her.

However, if your baby is still crying after you have fed, changed, and cuddled her, it is possible that air trapped in her stomach may be causing her discomfort.

Positions for burping

Put your baby over your shoulder and very gently pat or rub her back, making sure that you drape her well over the top of your shoulder with her arms hanging down your back. By doing this you are lengthening her trunk so that the wind can escape more readily. If your baby likes to spend a lot of time like this, it is a good idea to try to alternate shoulders, so that you don't get a stiff, aching neck on one side.

Another traditional burping position is to hold your baby with one hand open across her chest, supporting her head at the chin with your wide open thumb and index finger. Lean your baby slightly forward from the hips while straightening and

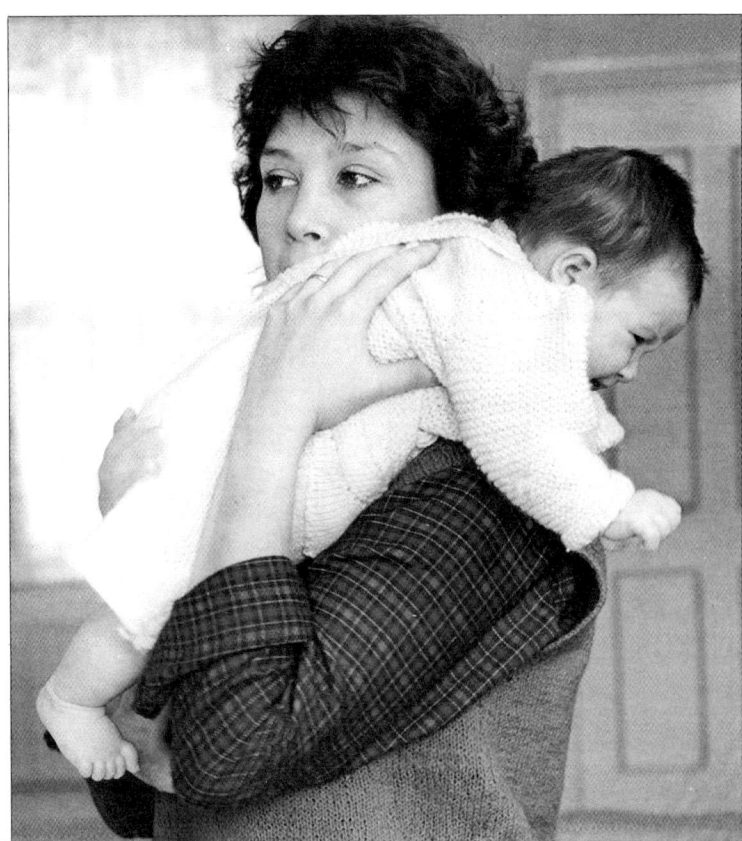

You can soothe or burp your baby by holding her over your shoulder so the trunk is elongated, then gently rub the back with your free hand.

lengthening her trunk with the supporting hand. At the same time gently rub or pat her back. As your baby may bring back a mouthful of food with the gas bubble, it is a good idea to protect your clothes with a diaper or towel.

Do not continue trying to burp your baby for too long – a couple of minutes is plenty. Any gas that is going to escape from the stomach will do so in this time, so if she continues to cry, try to think of the other possible reasons for her unhappiness.

"Three-month colic"

If you find that your baby is fretful and tense over a period of a few days at a regular time, particularly the evening, and that in spite of running through all the possible causes of discomfort she is still difficult to pacify for more than a few minutes, you may suspect that colic is the cause. Parents find this distressing

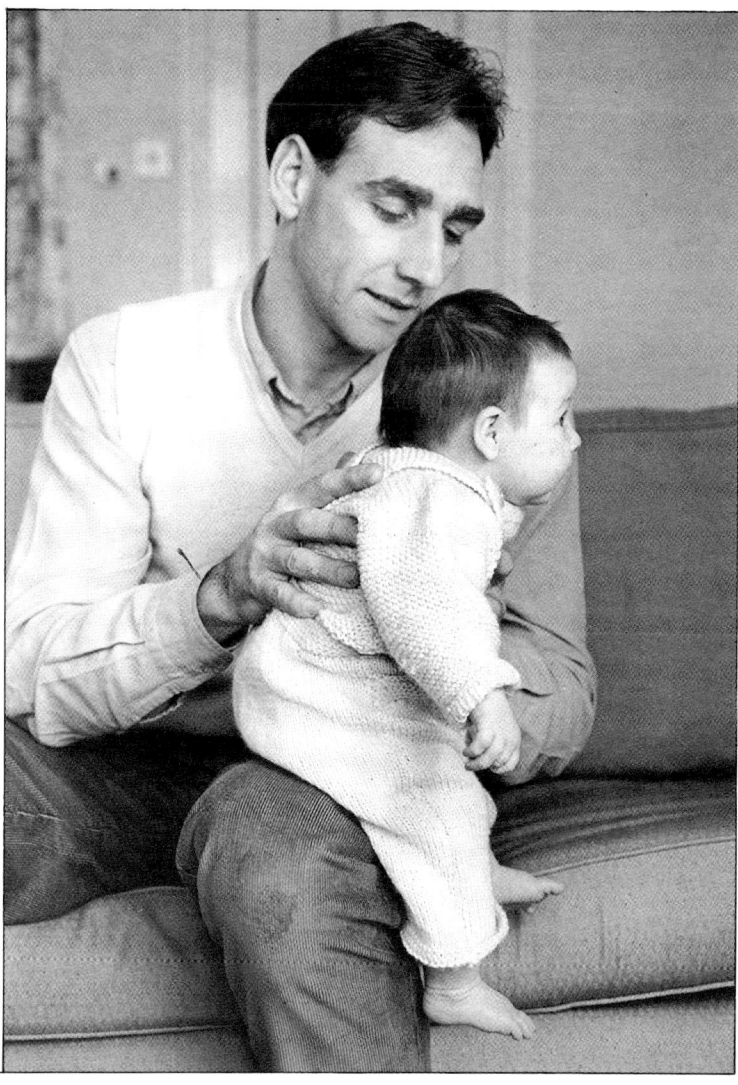

The baby's father can help by taking over at the end of the feeding to do the burping and changing.

problem very wearing, but babies generally grow out of this phase by about three months. Discuss it with your pediatrician. Frequent burping, even if the baby does not show any discomfort, will slow the baby's gulping, reducing the amount of air taken, thus preventing colic. Holding the baby along your arm (see page 65) may also help to relieve any colicky discomfort because it is an excellent position for bringing up gas.

Pacifiers

Many babies in their first three months have a strong urge to suck almost constantly. After a good feed, it is not hunger they are seeking to satisfy when they latch onto a breast, a teat, or a finger – they are sucking for comfort. An orthodontic pacifier will usually help during those miserable evening hours, or between feedings during the day. You can stop offering it to her

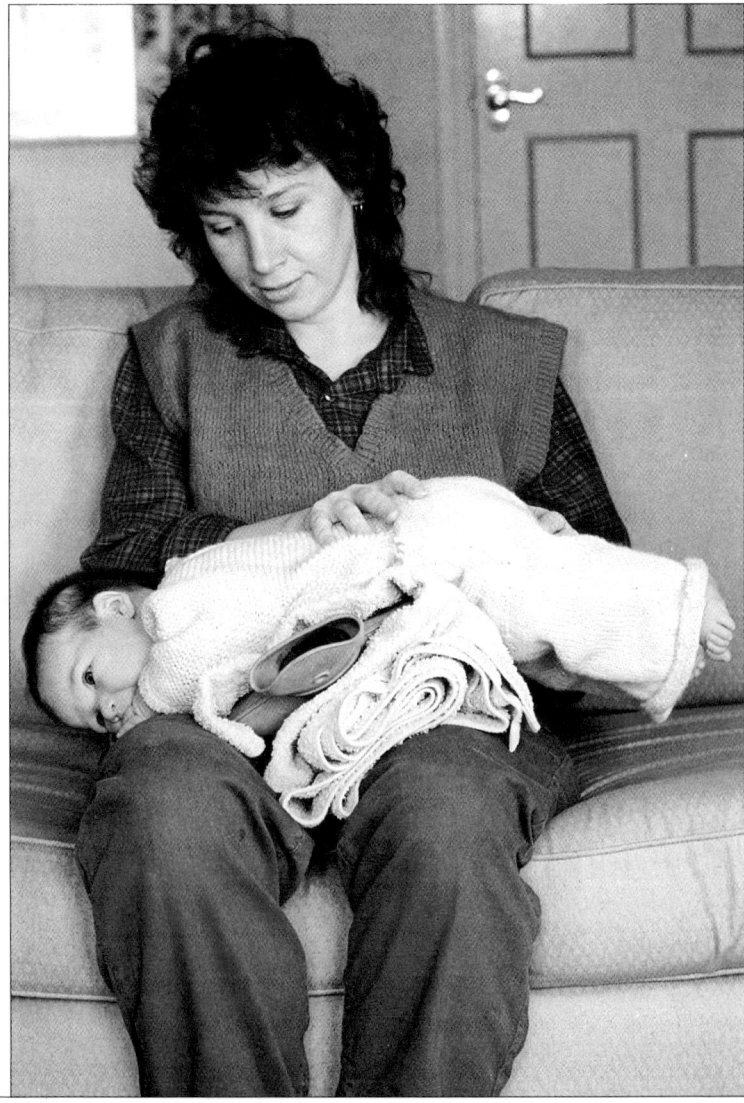

A restless baby can often be soothed in this position. The warmth of a wrapped hot water bottle under the stomach and the comfort of a hand on the back will often send the baby to sleep at last.

when she is three to five months old, or more settled, and before she becomes dependent on it. If you are prejudiced against using a pacifier, remind yourself firstly that it is preferable to the sound of a crying baby, and secondly that it is merely a crisis measure, until she becomes less dependent on sucking and more interested in her surroundings.

Baby massage

Most of us enjoy the soothing effect of gentle massage, and babies seem to be no exception. Choose a time when the baby is warm, comfortable, and well fed if you want to enjoy a massage with her. A little talcum powder or pure oil on the skin will help your hand movements, which should be smooth and slow with gentle pressure. Stroking downward along the length of the chest and abdomen or back with one hand or two will give both of you pleasure. The baby will probably also enjoy downward stroking along the arms and legs and gentle kneading of the soles of the feet with your thumbs. This baby massage, long used in the East, is thought to enhance a baby's feeling of well-being. But it should not become another chore for you. Even if you don't have time for a regular session, you are probably stroking and massaging your baby's skin every time you change a diaper or give a bath.

Sleeping, comfort, and safety

Recent research has shown that lying on the abdomen and overheating are two of the many factors thought to contribute to an increased risk of crib death. In the early weeks, therefore, a baby is often safer and happier lying on her side or back. After a while she will prefer to be less restricted. By the time she can roll voluntarily (around six to seven months) she will have decided for herself whether she likes to be on her front or back. Don't worry if she likes her front; a well baby of this age is perfectly safe in this position.

Portable beds and car seats

As your back is very vulnerable, weight and size should be considered when you make your choice of her first bed; a bassinet or cradle is light and easy to manage, but as it is not rigid it must not be used in a car. If you want to use a portable bed in the back seat of a car, it must have a rigid frame and be secured by restrainer straps. Make sure your baby's heavy head is always carried nearest you as you lift the bassinet. The safest way for your baby to travel in a car is in a rear-facing car seat, held in place by an adult seat belt; this provides protection for your baby in the event of an accident. Choose one that is light, has handles, is easy to transport, and meets federal safety guidelines; it is perfectly safe for newborn babies and should be used to take your baby home from the hospital. *Never* hold your baby, toddler, or child on your lap during a car trip—it is much too dangerous!

A mother often finds that one of the easiest ways to keep herself and her baby happy is to drive to see a friend; her baby falls asleep in the car seat and when she arrives she is free to enjoy adult conversation. Unfortunately, car seats are not ideal beds. Once the motion of the car has stopped, babies tend merely to

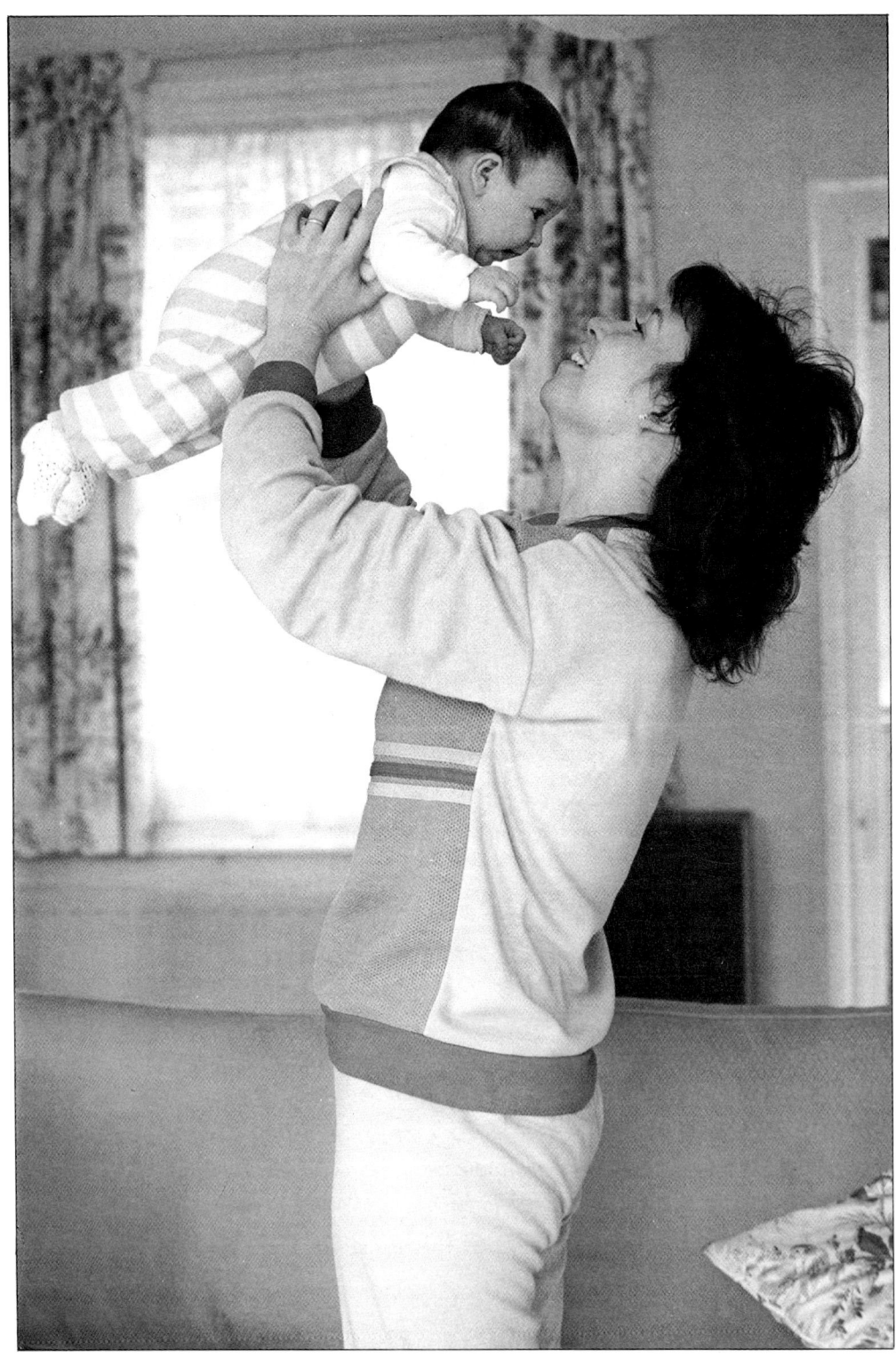

"catnap" and a day passed largely in a car seat will probably irritate and unsettle your baby. So try to provide one or two hours in the morning and afternoon when your young baby can lie flat and sleep if she wishes, wherever you may be.

Baby carriages

Remember when choosing a baby carriage the handle height should be somewhere between your hip bone and waist. Most mothers find a carriage indispensable in the first few months, and for many babies it is their first bed. By gently rocking the carriage or taking them out for a walk in it, their parents find they are guaranteed almost certain peace. Parents who also have a young toddler can harness the older child to a special seat on the front of the carriage, while piling the shopping into the basket underneath. This way the baby is lulled to sleep, the toddler is taken for an outing, and parents bring home all their shopping with no strain to their backs. Of course, the children cannot be left unattended, even for a moment, since the extra weight of a lively toddler can cause even the sturdiest carriage to tilt.

Mother and baby medical examinations

Six weeks is the traditional time for a new mother's postnatal examination, but you and your body may need longer to recover from childbirth. Your uterus should have returned to its pre-pregnancy shape and size, you will probably notice that you have better control of your abdominal muscles, and the acute pain from your stitches will have faded. Your baby will probably be rewarding you by this time with wonderful smiles, have established a fairly regular feeding pattern, and have better control of the head. It is for all these reasons that four to six weeks is generally chosen as the ideal time for a doctor to check both of you.

Your postnatal checkup

It is very important to make an appointment with your obstetrician for a checkup after four to six weeks. A blood test may be done to see if you are anemic, and your blood pressure will be taken. Your doctor will want to check that your uterus has fully involuted, give you a vaginal examination, and check your pelvic floor muscles. The doctor should also examine your breasts, whether you are breastfeeding or not, and take a cervical smear for testing if you have not had one within the last year. Now is the time to discuss any postnatal problems such as bladder leakage, backache, painful intercourse, or persistent depression. It is also important to talk about methods of contraception.

Your baby's first checkup

You will probably have visited your pediatrician before this, but at six weeks the doctor will give your baby a thorough checkup to monitor progress. The doctor will record his weight, measure his length and head and chest circumference; look at his eye movements; check his response to sound; and ask you if the baby has begun to smile. The doctor will also examine the hips and genitals, feel the abdomen, listen to the heart sounds and lung expansion, and check the head control when pulled up to sitting. Don't be afraid to mention anything about your baby that is worrying you, however insignificant it may seem.

Six weeks after the birth is a good time to assess the progress of both mother and baby.

MAKING PROGRESS

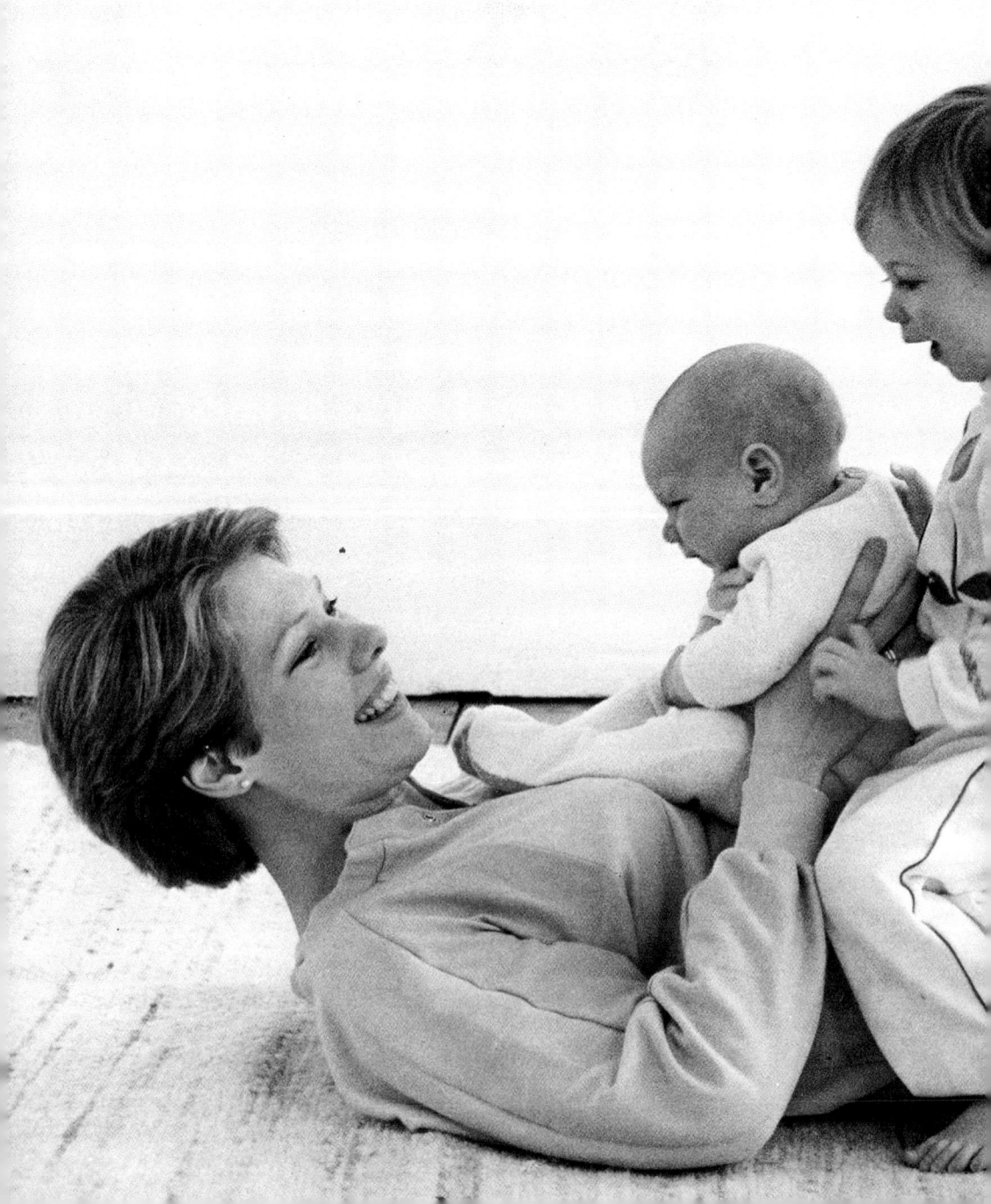

EXERCISES
6 WEEKS TO
3 MONTHS

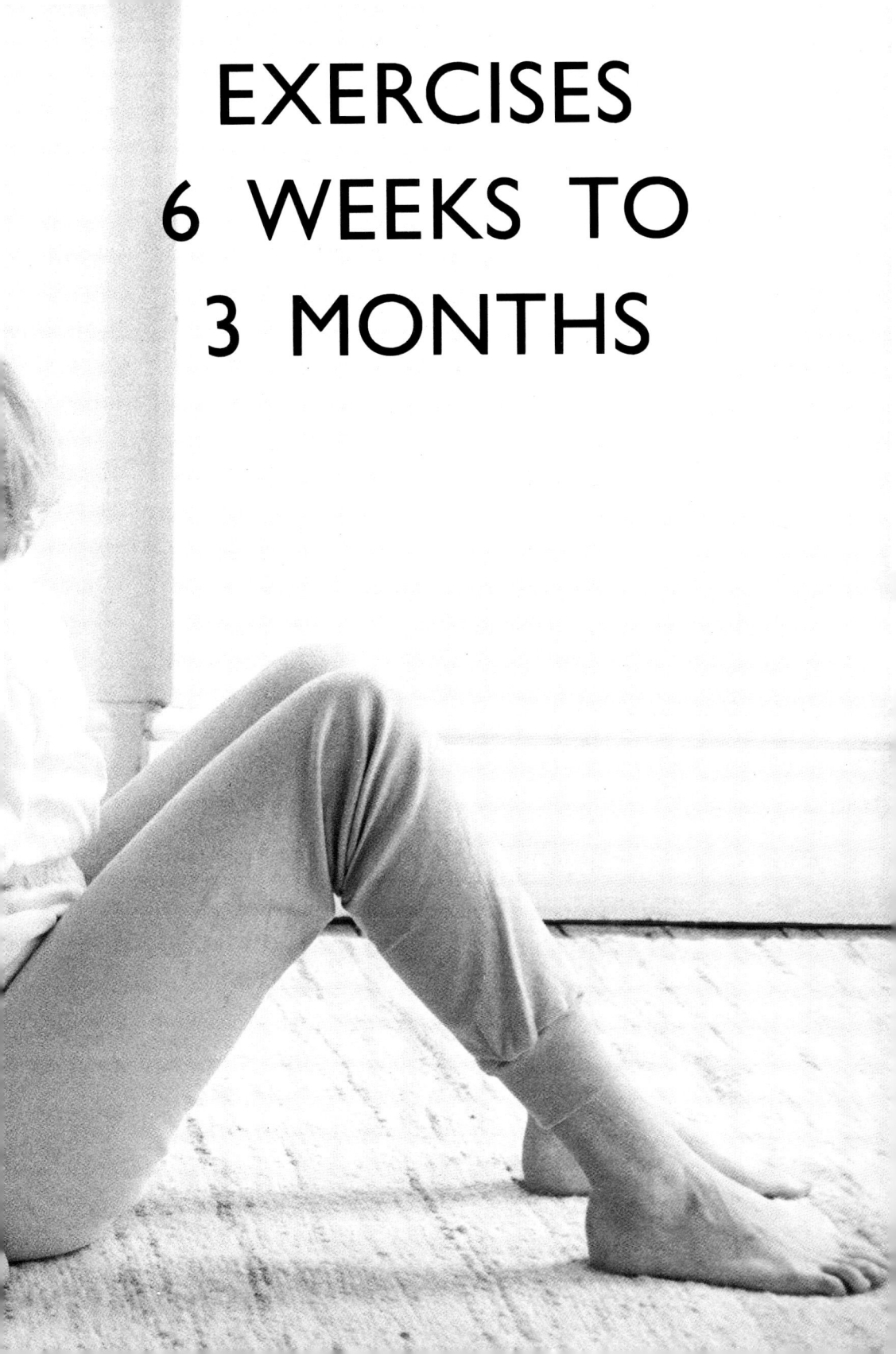

By now your baby may have begun to establish a routine and will not be so dependent on you for contact when he wakes. You may also be beginning to adjust to the pattern of broken nights and the extra chores and will be able to devote more time and energy to your postnatal recovery.

You will probably find by now that your baby is beginning to respond to being moved and handled, becoming less passive and enjoying simple games and activities to help stimulate development. As the baby is now more alert and has some head control, you can put him near you as you exercise, or even let him join in.

Your ligaments are now stronger and firmer but have by no means fully recovered. Continue to take care when bending, twisting, and lifting since they can still be easily damaged.

Your muscles will have regained some of their strength and you should be ready to move on to stronger and more difficult exercises. You can begin these earlier if you feel ready. Usually though, and especially after your first baby, it takes quite a while to become used to an entirely different life-style, and exercises often have to take second or third place on your list of priorities!

Feeding exercises

Continue using feeding times to tone and strengthen your abdominal and pelvic floor muscles. Make sure that you tighten and relax the muscles of the perineum at least twenty times or more per feeding. You should now be aiming to hold each pelvic floor "squeeze" for up to eight seconds. To strengthen the muscles as much as possible, you should try to increase the power of each contraction for the last three to four seconds like this: pull your pelvic floor muscles in and up, hold it – 2, 3, 4, 5 – now increase the squeeze – *more, more, more*, and then relax. Also spend a few moments on your abdominal muscles, holding them in firmly for eight to ten counts while continuing to breathe naturally.

Strengthening exercises

You should also try to set aside a short time twice a day to concentrate on stronger ways of working these groups of muscles, while adding new exercises for your back, buttocks, and legs, plus your chest and arm muscles.

Aerobic exercise

Besides a regular program of strengthening exercises, some form of brisk aerobic exercise, which burns up oxygen and fat and increases your heart rate, is important. To help lose weight you need to do this at least three times a week. A brisk, long walk in the fresh air is the easiest and cheapest form of vigorous exercise. If your toddler slows you down, let him/her enjoy a leisurely stroll before being put in the carriage or stroller. Swimming is another excellent method of burning up fat and improving your fitness; you can begin as soon as your lochia (postpartum vaginal discharge) has ceased. Walking, swimming, and exercising with friends will improve your social life as well as your body.

LYING ON THE FLOOR

STATIC PELVIC CONTRACTIONS

This exercise helps firm your abdomen and buttocks and strengthens your pelvic floor.

Lie on the floor with your knees bent; your baby can sit on your stomach. Draw your pelvic floor muscles inward and upward, concentrating on your vagina. Hold on hard and then contract your buttocks so that your bottom lifts up off the floor. Blow out, pulling in your abdomen, and lift your head so that your baby can see your face. Hold for four counts, then lower slowly, relaxing all the working muscles. Start with six lifts, then progress to twenty and also increase the length of time from four to ten counts.

If you still find it difficult to *feel* your pelvic floor working, it may be helpful after a bath to insert two fingers into your vagina while you stand with one foot on the edge of the bathtub. Now squeeze your pelvic floor muscles. You should feel them tightening against your fingers. Constant practice improves your power. Consult your doctor if you are worried about your pelvic floor muscle or bladder control.

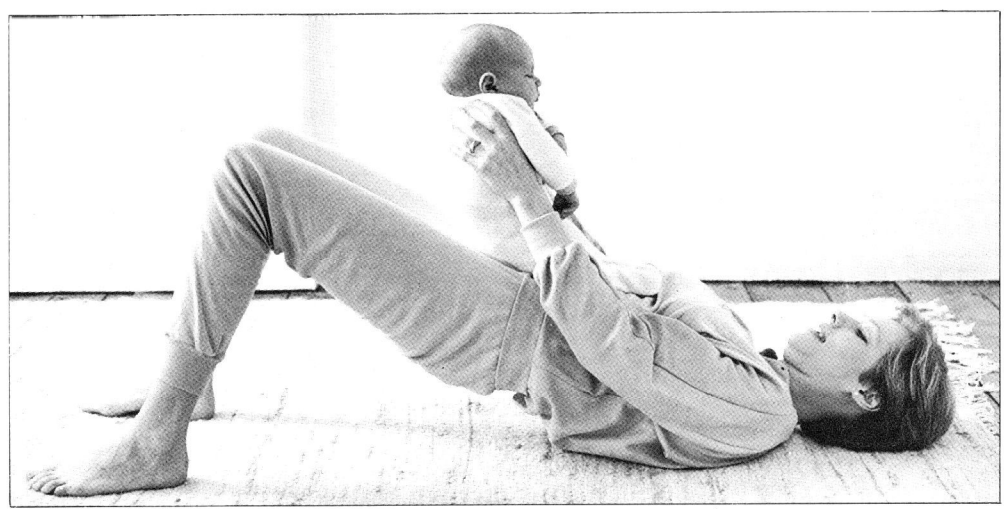

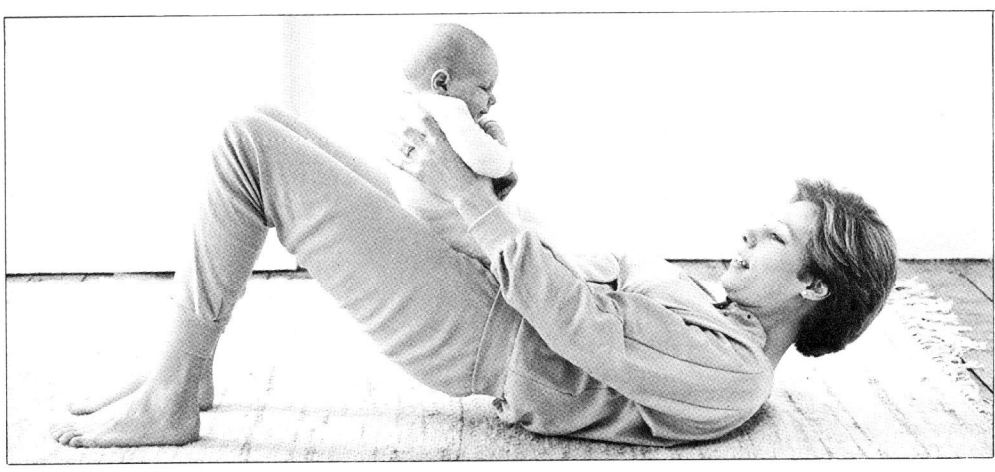

SIT-UPS OR CRUNCHES

This strong exercise will help firm your vertical abdominal muscles and draw them closer together.

Lie on your back with your knees bent up high and your hands on your thighs. Tilt your pelvis by pulling in your abdominal muscles and drawing your buttocks together at the same time. Tuck your chin in, blow out, and slowly curl your head and shoulders up off the floor, pushing your hands along your thighs toward your knees. Hold this position for four counts and then lower yourself slowly back to the floor. Do this six times and increase to twenty.

You can increase the length of time you hold the curled-up position, and if you cross your arms over your chest, or put your hands behind your head when you curl up, the exercise will be even more challenging.

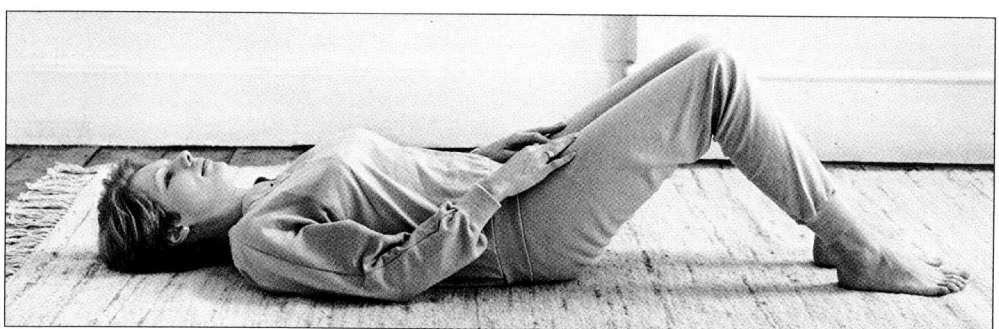

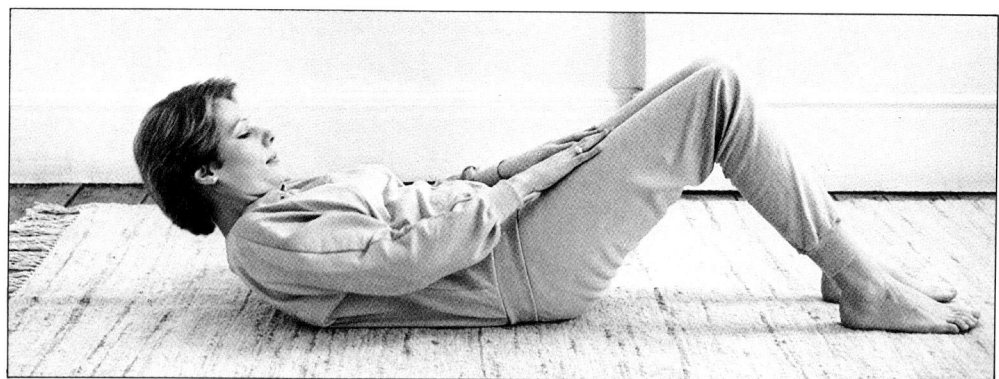

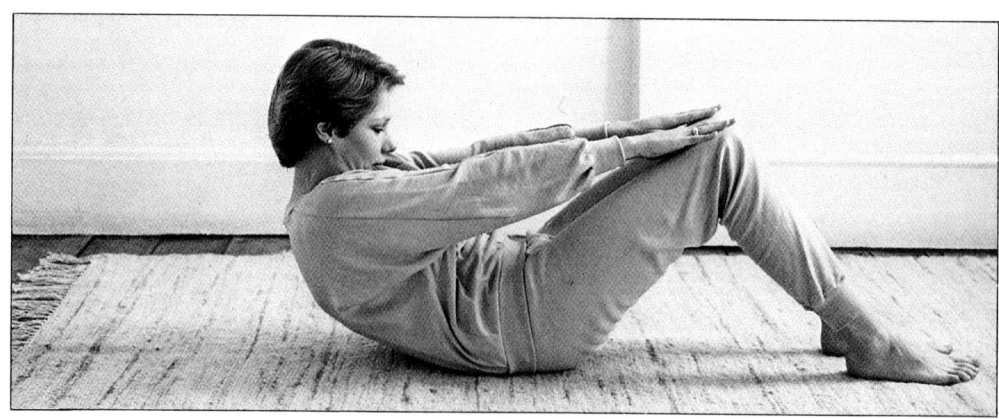

LATERAL LEG TWISTS

This exercise uses your oblique abdominal and lower back muscles to slim your waist.

Lie on the floor with your arms away from your sides, your knees bent up high, and your feet flat. Pull in your abdominal muscles, then move your knees to the left, until your thigh touches the floor. Keeping your knees tightly together and your abdomen firmly in, move your knees to the right and then back to the middle; pause, then repeat. It is important to keep both shoulders flat on the floor as you roll your legs from side to side and *very* important to remember to hold in your abdominal muscles throughout the exercise.

Start with six and increase to twenty times, progressing the exercise by omitting the pause and increasing the speed of the movement. You may find it helpful to put your hands under your head when you speed up this exercise.

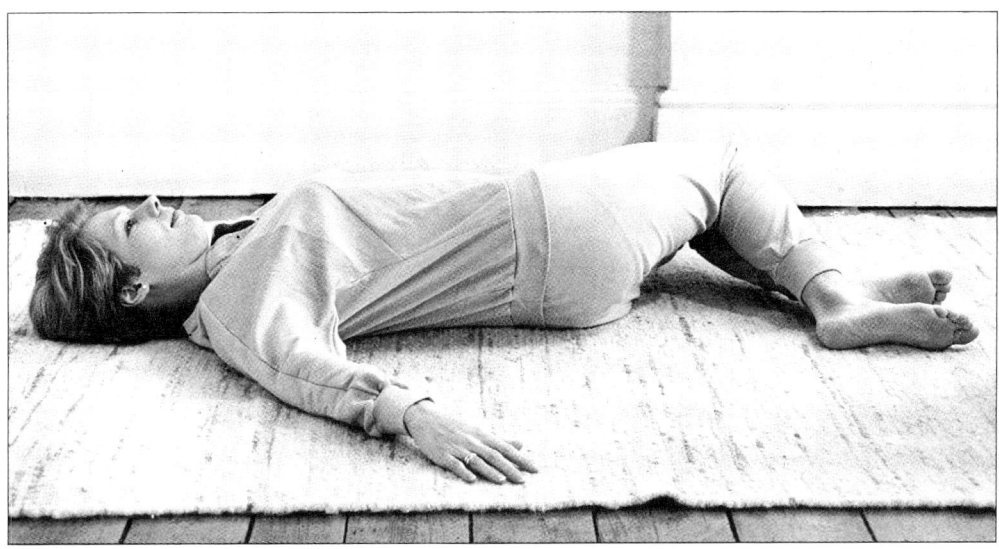

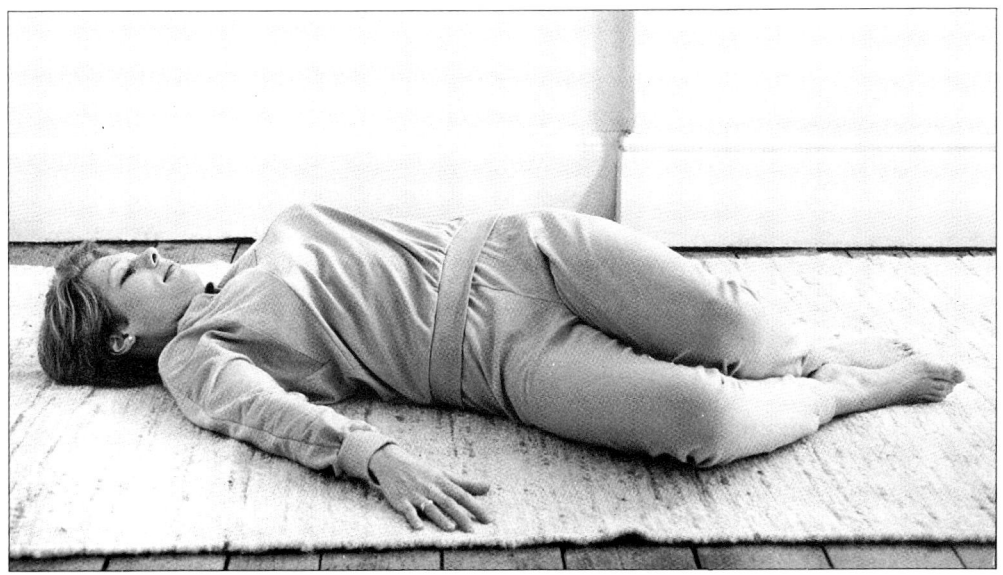

LATERAL SIT-UPS (LATERAL CRUNCHES)

This exercise uses both sets of oblique abdominal muscles and helps slim the waist. Lie on the floor, knees bent up high, and your arms by your sides. Pull in your stomach firmly and hold it there. Blow out and stretch your right hand toward your left foot, twisting at the waist. Hold this position for four counts and then lower back again. Repeat with your left hand stretching toward your right foot. You will not be able to reach your foot at first, but gradually you will get closer. Start with six on each side, and increase to twenty.

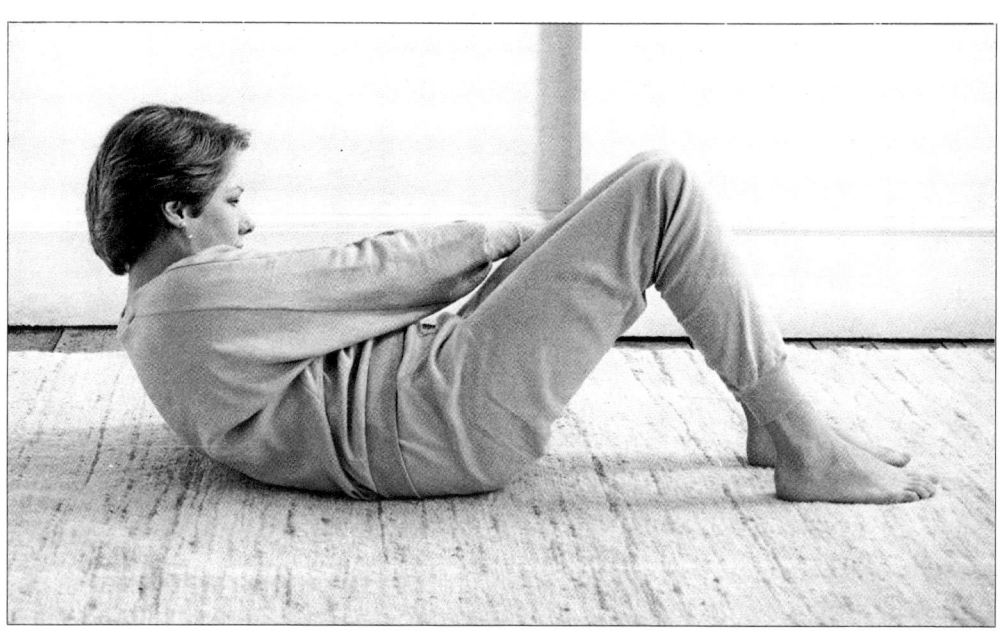

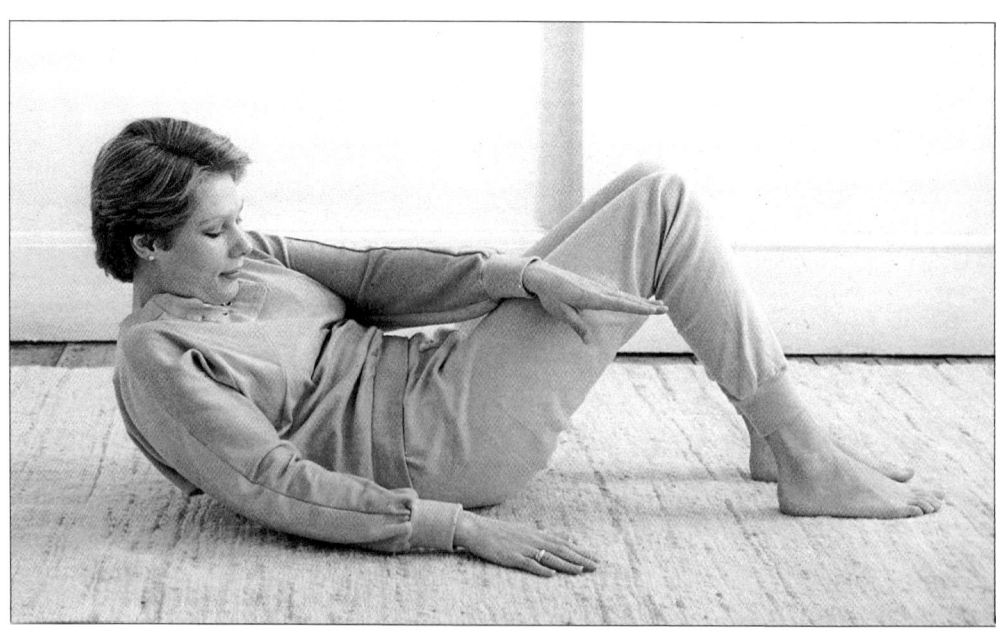

LATERAL BENDS — SUPINE

This exercise will help to flatten your stomach and slim your waist.

Lie on your back with your knees bent up high. Pull your abdomen in firmly and hold it there. Blow out and slide your right hand down toward your right foot, side-bending from your waist, then, still holding in your abdomen, come back to the middle. Relax, breathing easily, then repeat to the left. Start with six to each side and increase to twenty.

It is most important to make sure that you continue holding in your abdomen during the movements. This exercise can be progressed by omitting the pause between bending to the right and left, and making the movement continuous and faster.

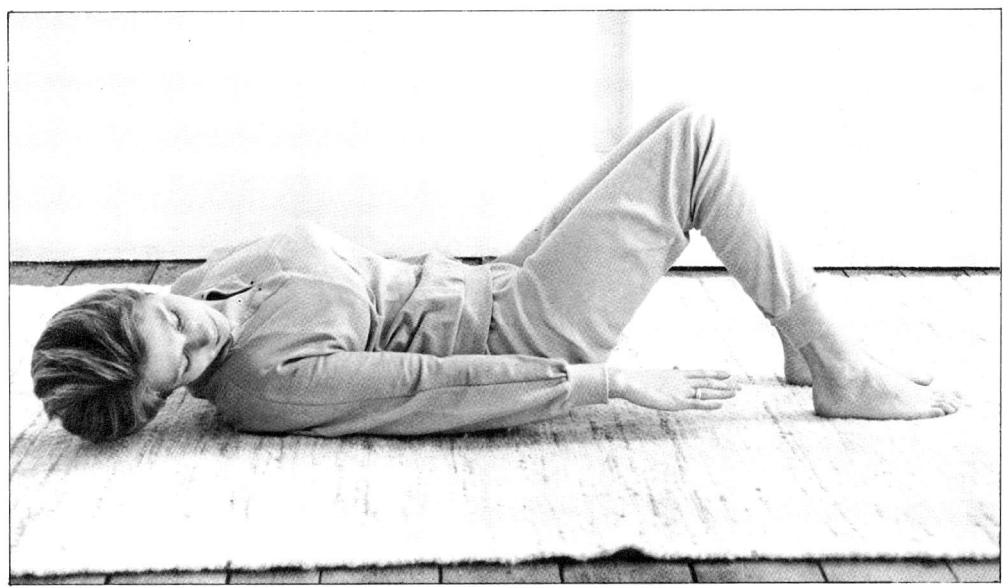

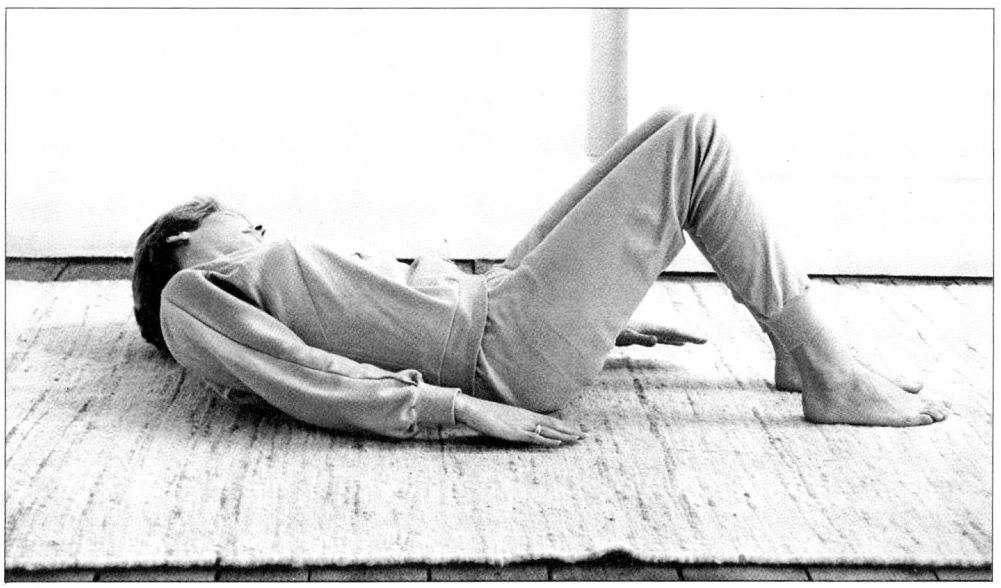

LEG ABDUCTIONS

Lie on your right side, resting your head on your right hand with your left hand on the floor in front of you. Pull your abdominal muscles in firmly and hold them there. Lift your left leg straight up sideways as high as you can, without letting it stray forward or backward. Hold it there for four counts and then lower. Repeat, lying on your left side. Do this six times each side, increasing to twenty. This exercise can be made harder by not allowing your leg to go all the way down between lifts.

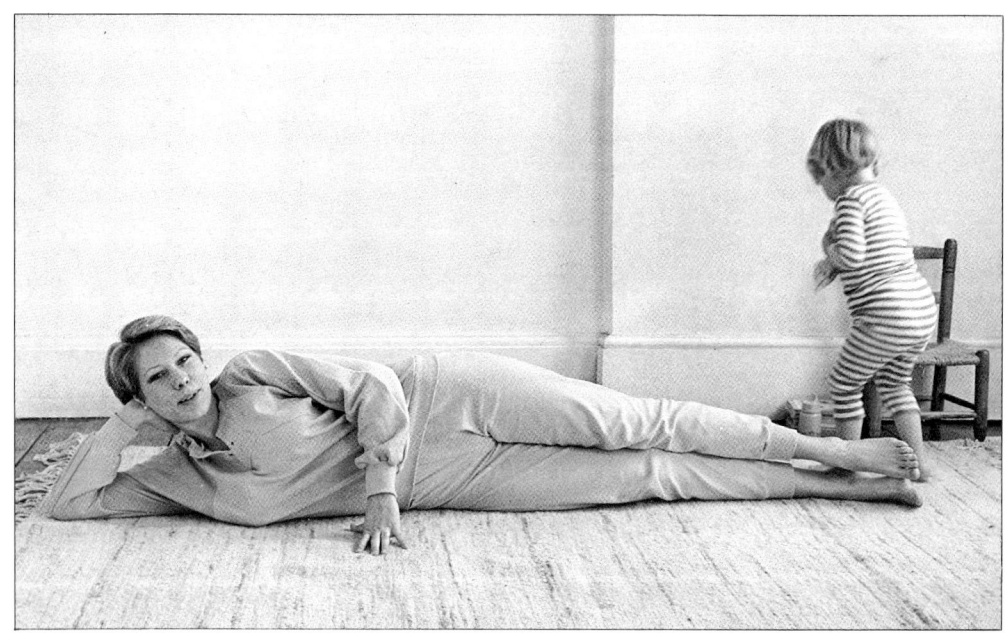

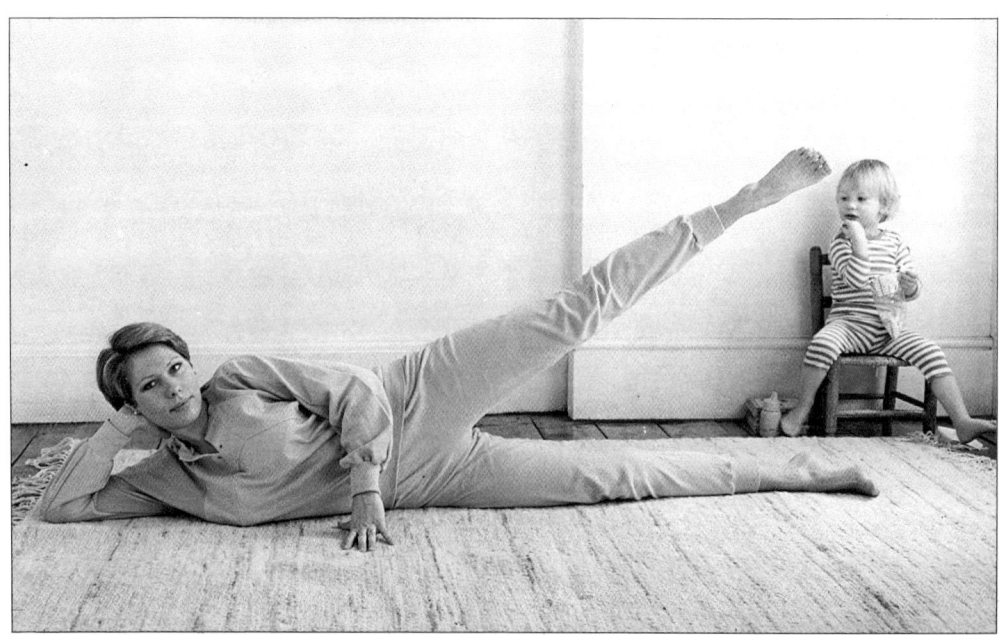

BUTTOCK FIRMER AND BACK STRENGTHENER

This exercise tightens and strengthens your buttocks and lower back muscles.

Lie on your front and rest your head on your hands. Pull your buttocks tightly together and then lift both straight legs, knees pressed tightly together, as high as you can off the floor. Hold for four counts and lower slowly. Start with six and increase to twenty-four. Remember to breathe normally. If you experience back pain during or after this exercise, leave it out; but continue doing the Prone Leg Hyperextensions (page 61).

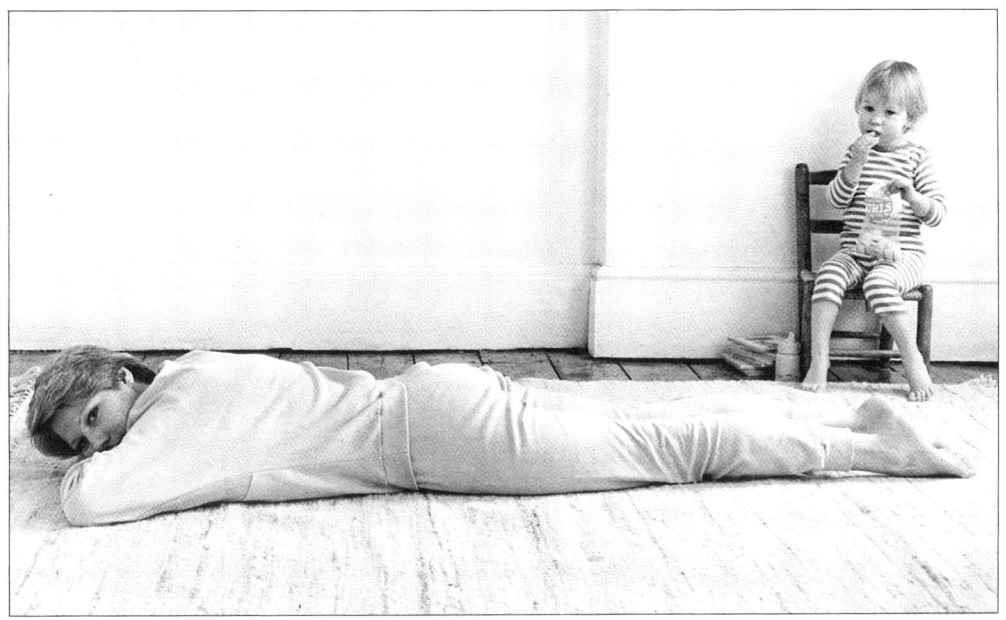

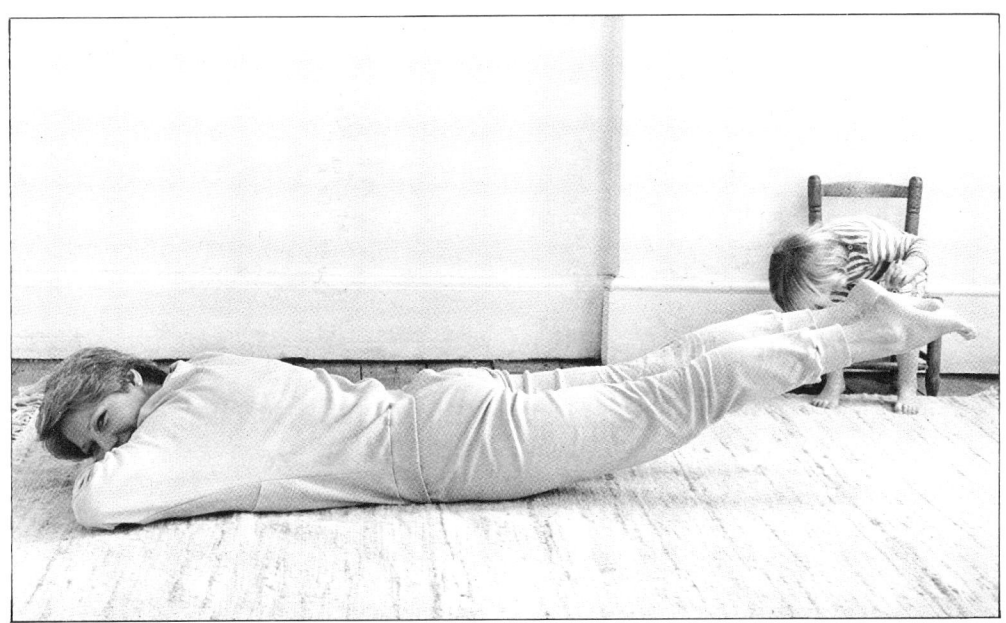

SITTING ON THE FLOOR

NEGATIVE SIT-UPS

This works your straight abdominal muscles hard.

Sit up straight with your knees bent up high and both arms stretched out in front of you. Tilt up your pubic bone by holding your abdominal and buttock muscles in firmly. Keeping your back rounded, blow out and curl your body downward toward the floor. When you reach half way, stop and hold this position for four counts, breathing normally, then slowly sit up. Start with six and increase to twenty.

To progress this exercise, hold the "down-curled" position a little longer, continuing to breathe normally. Progress further by putting your hands behind your head.

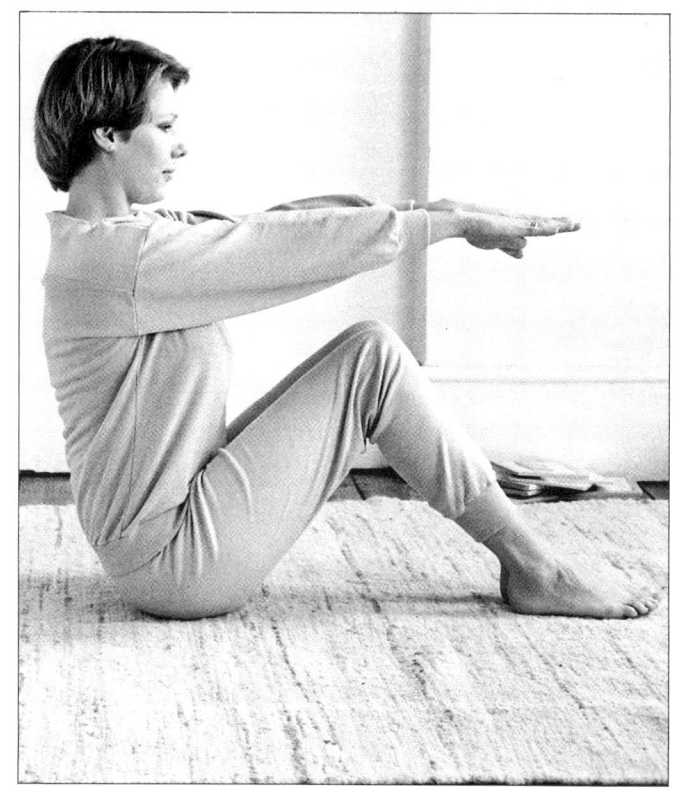

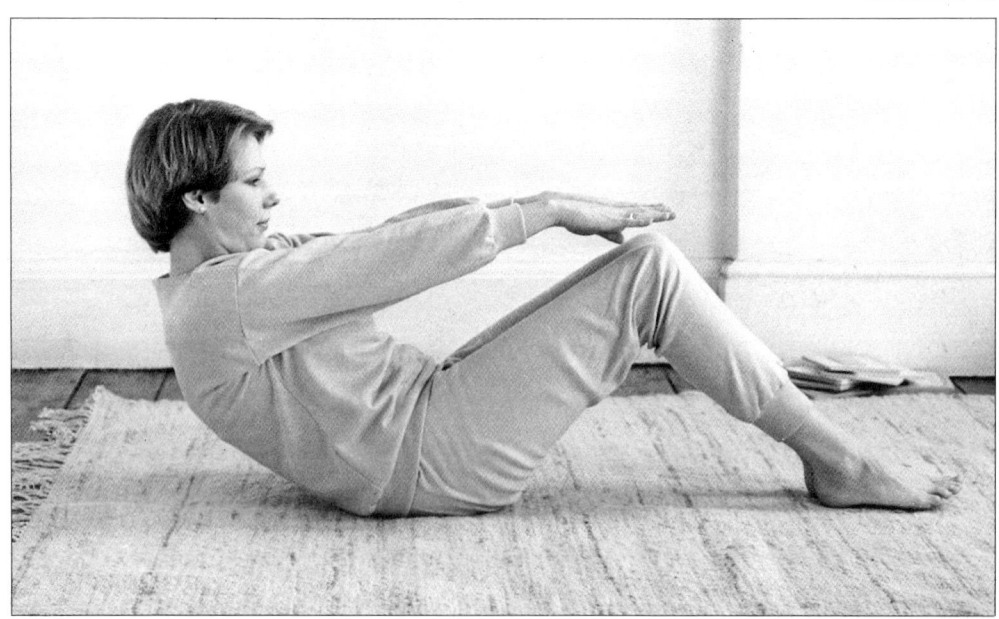

BOTTOM-WALKING

This exercise strengthens your back, abdominal, and thigh muscles, as well as slimming your waist.

Sit on the floor with your back straight and both legs and arms stretched in front of you. "Walk" forward on your bottom, keeping your abdominal muscles pulled in tightly at the same time. Take eight "steps" forward and eight backward. Remember to keep your back tall and straight and your stomach well pulled in as you move. Start with six sequences and increase to twenty. Your baby may enjoy sitting on your lap while you do this exercise.

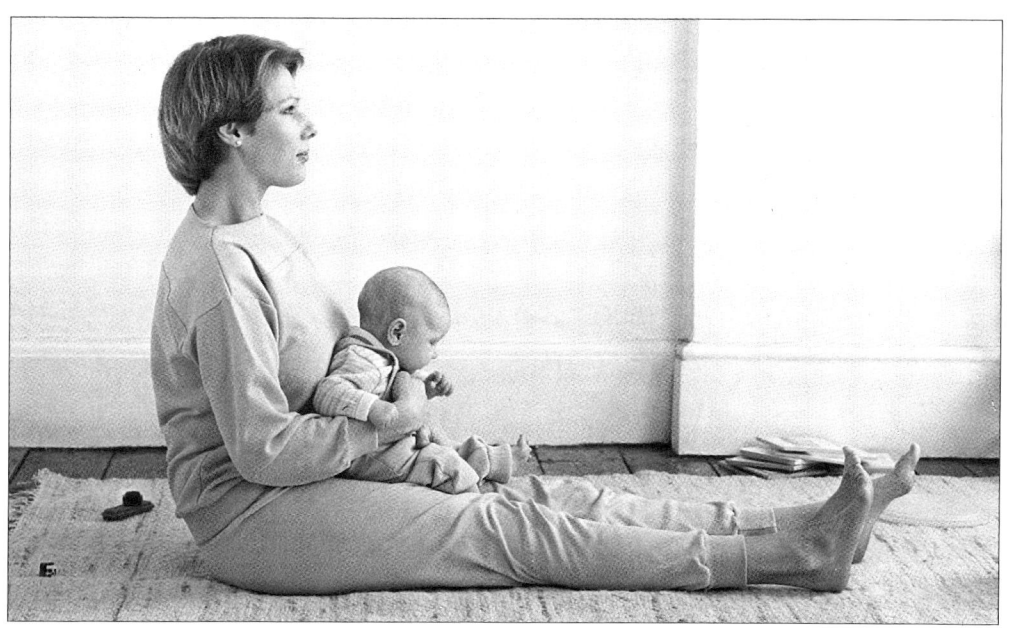

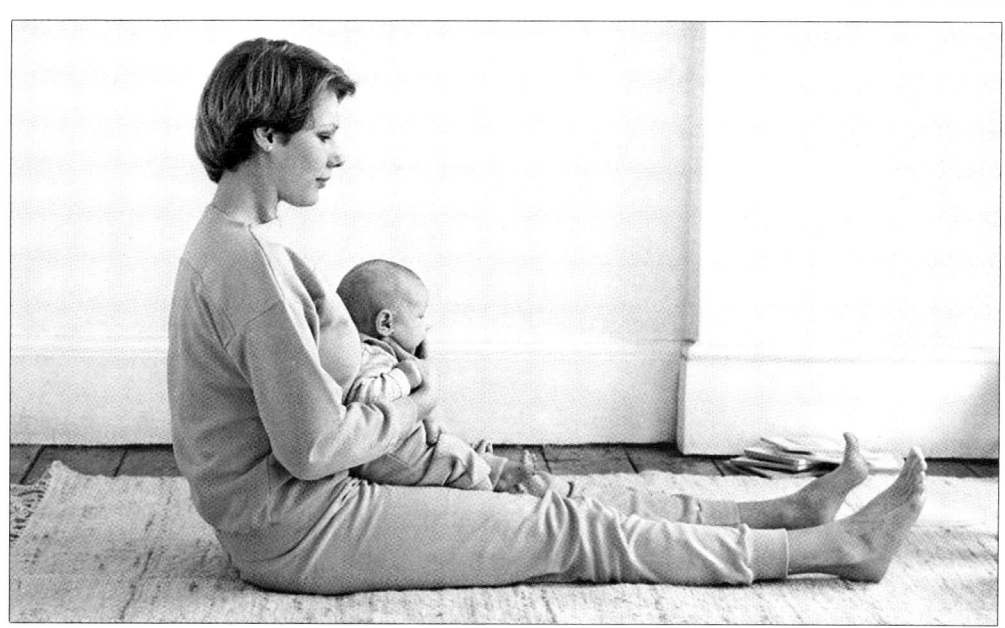

ON ALL FOURS

CAT ARCH

In this exercise you are working your abdominal muscles against gravity. When you are on all fours, you will notice that your stomach really sags when you relax, but when you tighten your muscles to rock your pelvis you can make it quite flat again. This exercise not only strengthens your abdominal muscles but also your buttocks, and it may help to ease an aching back.

Kneel on all fours, with your baby lying on the floor below you so that you can look at one another. Blow out, and arch your back by tucking in your abdominal and buttock muscles so that your pubic bone moves forward. Hold for four counts, then gently relax your muscles so that your back is flat again. Feel the rocking of your pelvis and the muscles that work to do it. Repeat ten times, increasing to twenty.

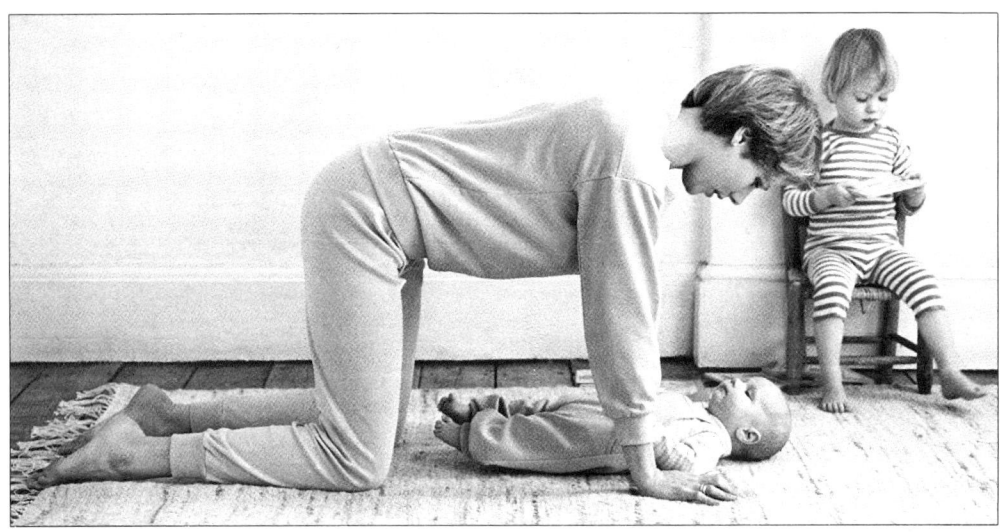

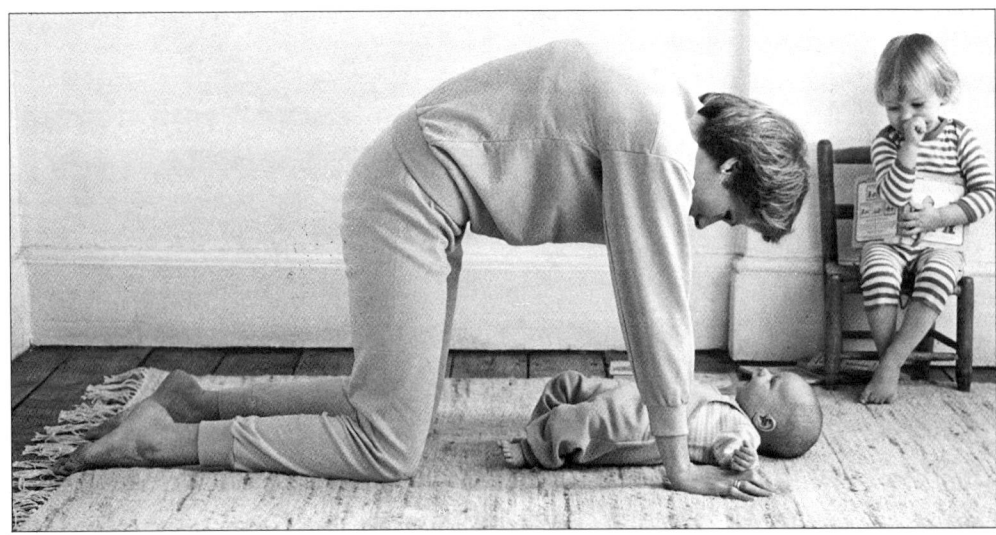

LATERAL LOOKS

This exercise strengthens the abdominal muscles at your front and sides, helping to reduce your waistline. Kneel on all fours and pull in your abdominal muscles to flatten your stomach. Turn your head to the right and bend at the waist so you can see your right hip. Return to the middle and relax. Repeat the process on the left side, alternating ten times and then increasing to twenty. Now drop the pause between each side and briskly "wag" your bottom from side to side, with abdominal muscles well pulled in.

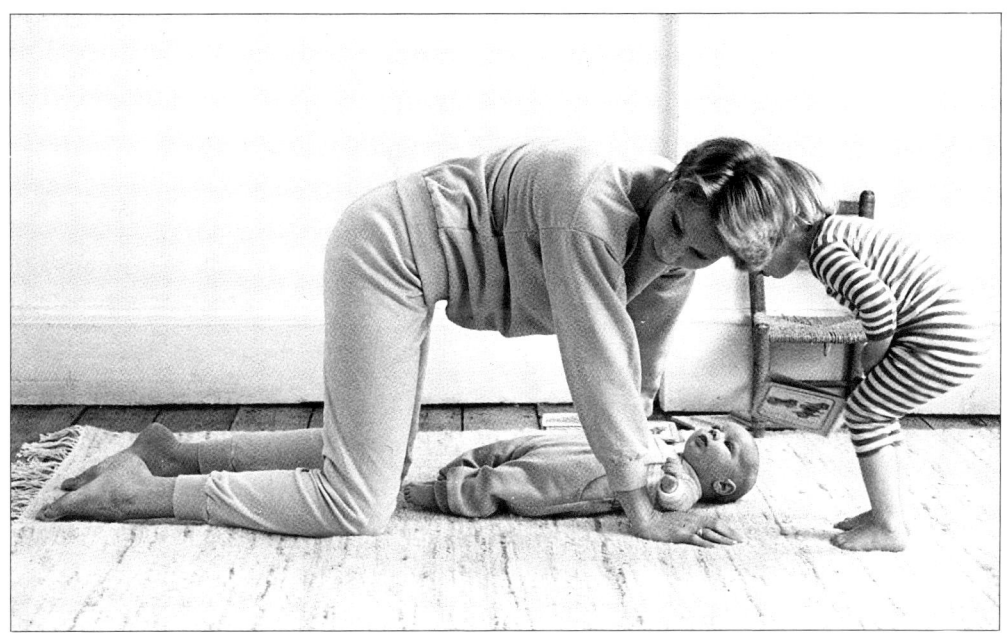

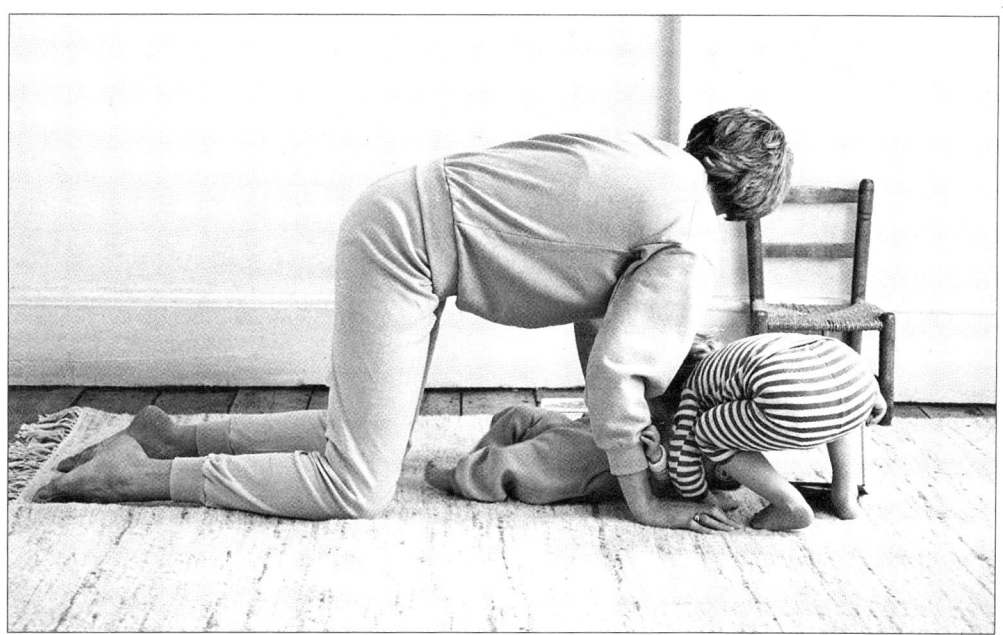

LEG KICKBACKS

This exercise will strengthen the back, abdominal, buttock, and thigh muscles.

Kneel comfortably on all fours – your baby may enjoy lying on the floor looking up at your face – now try to touch your right knee with your nose and pull your abdomen well in at the same time. Then stretch this leg out and up behind you, feeling your buttocks tighten as you hold the leg in place for four counts. Lower the leg, and repeat the movement on the other side. To start with, try doing this exercise six times on each side and increase it to twelve times.

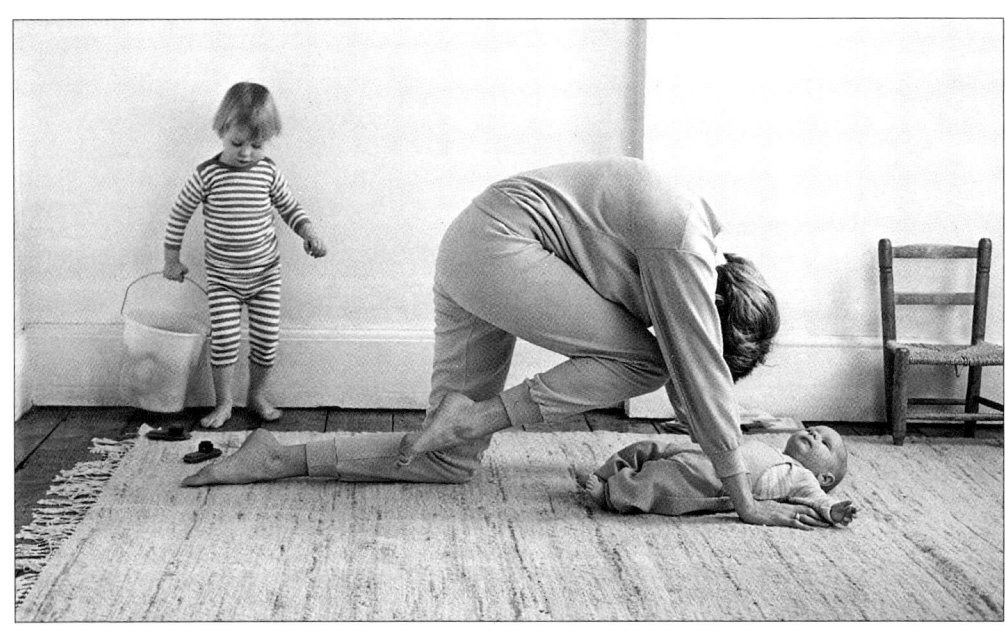

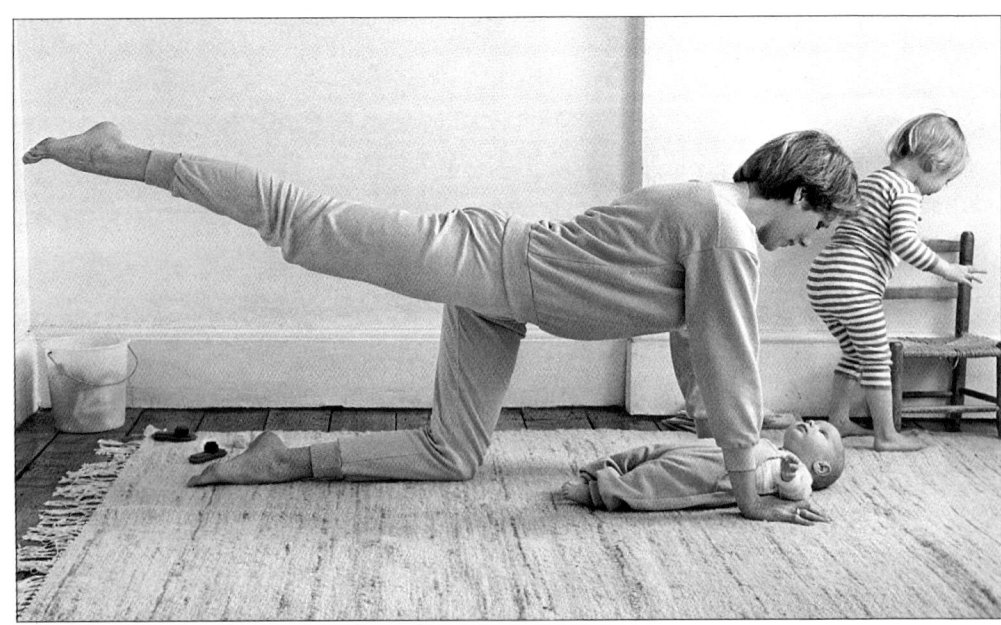

STANDING UP

WALL SITS

This simple exercise strengthens your postural muscles, firms your buttocks and abdomen, and shapes your thighs. Do it carefully if you have had knee problems and stop if you experience knee pains.

Hold your baby with his back resting on your chest, your forearm lying across one shoulder and his chest and stomach, with your hand supporting him between his legs. Stand with your back against the wall with your feet slightly apart and about 12–15 in (30–38 cm) from the wall. Pull in your abdominal muscles and squeeze your buttocks together, pressing your waist against the wall. Now, slowly bend your knees and slide 6–12 in (15 30 cm) down the wall, keeping your back firmly pressed against the wall from your waist upward all the time. Hold this position while you count slowly up to six, then gradually straighten your knees again. As you get stronger, you can increase the length of time you keep your knees bent – but not so long that the thigh muscles begin to tremble.

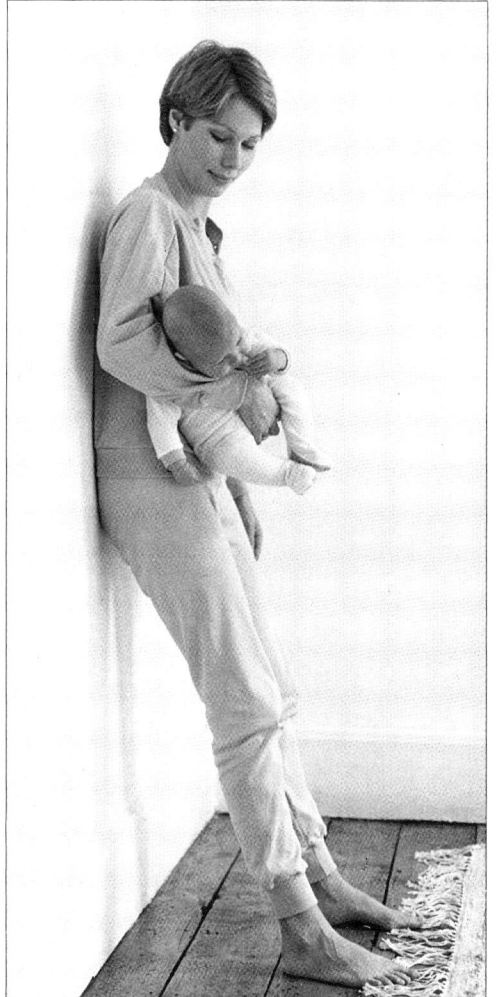
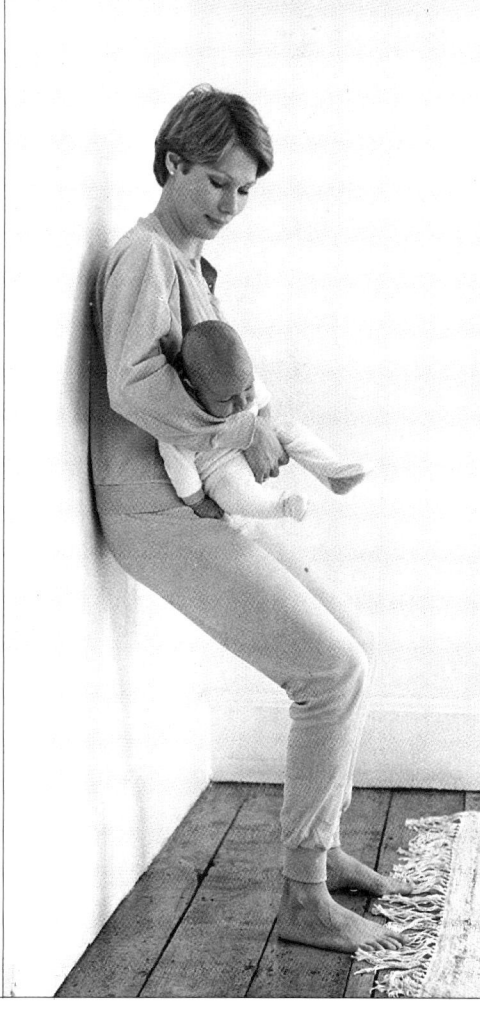

WALL PUSH-UPS

This exercise will strengthen and firm the muscles of your chest and upper arms. It will help you with all the lifting and carrying you will probably be doing by now, but is far less strenuous than regular floor push-ups.

Stand with your feet about 2 ft (60 cm) from the wall, and 1 ft (30 cm) apart. Lean your body weight on your hands, then, keeping your back and legs straight and in line, bend your elbows so that your face is almost touching the wall. Hold for four counts, then straighten your arms and push yourself back. Repeat the exercise ten times at first, gradually increasing it to twenty. You can work these arm and chest muscles harder by lying face downward, hands open on the floor just outside your shoulders and pushing your trunk upward, but, unlike regular floor push-ups, keeping your hips and thighs on the floor. Lower your trunk gently, then repeat slowly, ten times. Do not do this floor exercise if your back aches.

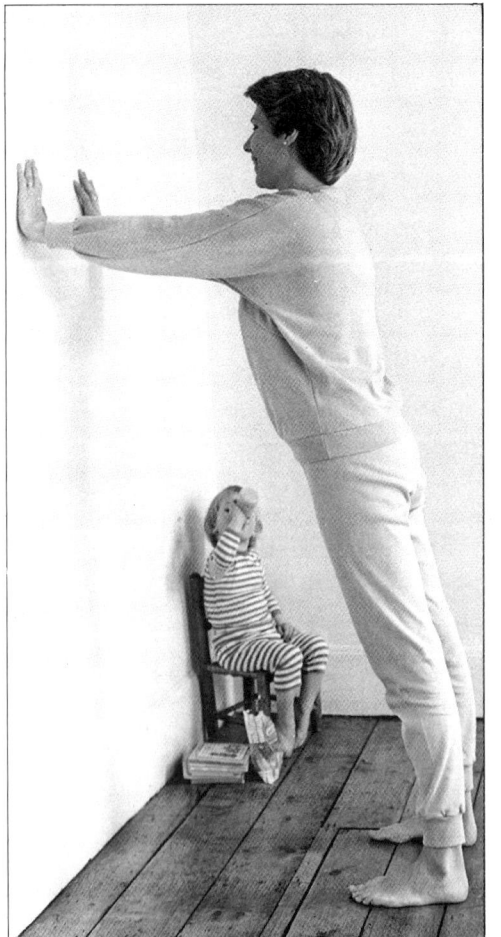
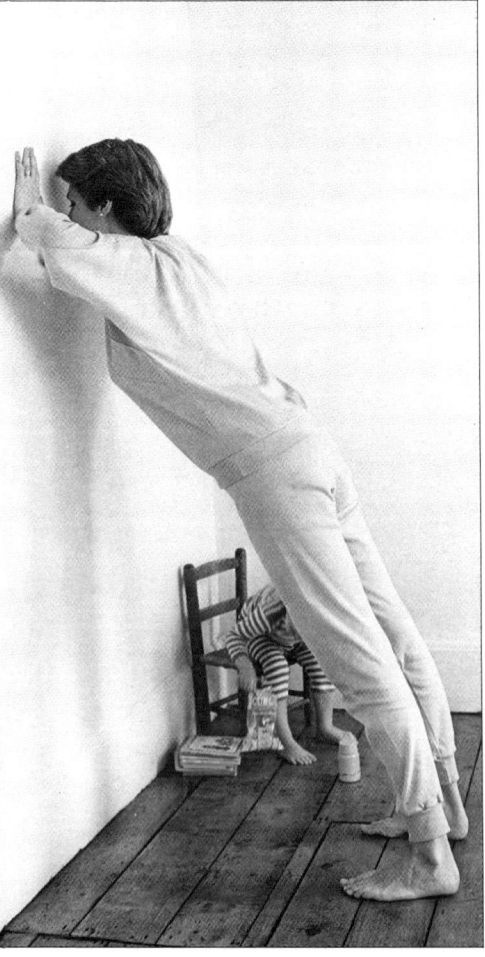

DAILY PROGRAM

Reminder Try to do these exercises the recommended number of times, twice a day. Asterisks mark the most important exercises, so on days when you have very little time, at least try to do these. Continue to contract your stomach and pelvic floor muscles during feedings.

Lying on the floor

*STATIC PELVIC CONTRACTIONS
Abdominal muscles, buttocks, pelvic floor
page 75   6 to 20 times

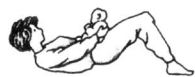

SIT-UPS OR CRUNCHES
Vertical abdominal muscles
page 76
6 to 20 times

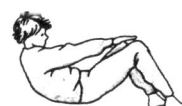

LATERAL LEG TWISTS
Abdominal and lower back muscles page 77
6 to 20 times

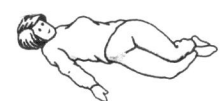

*LATERAL SIT-UPS (LATERAL CRUNCHES)
Oblique abdominal muscles page 78
6 to 20 times

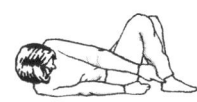

*LATERAL BENDS — SUPINE
Oblique and vertical abdominal muscles
page 79
6 to 20 times

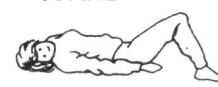

LEG ABDUCTIONS
Thighs and abdominal muscles
page 80
6 to 20 times

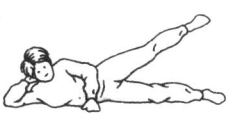

BUTTOCK FIRMER AND BACK STRENGTHENER
Buttocks and lower back muscles
page 81
6 to 24 times

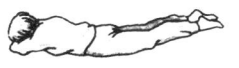

Sitting on the floor

*NEGATIVE SIT-UPS
Vertical abdominal muscles
page 82
6 to 20 times

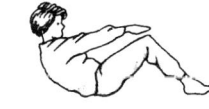

BOTTOM-WALKING
Back, abdominal, and thigh muscles
page 83
6 to 20 times

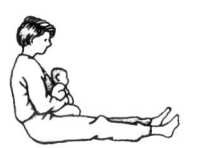

On all fours

CAT ARCH
Abdominal muscles, buttocks, and to ease backache page 84
10 to 20 times

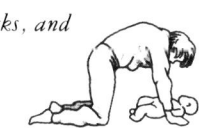

LATERAL LOOKS
Vertical and oblique abdominal muscles
page 85
10 to 20 times

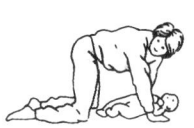

LEG KICKBACKS
Abdominal, back, buttock, and thigh muscles page 86
6 to 12 times

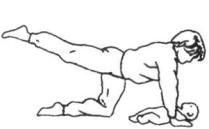

Standing up

WALL-SITS
Back muscles, buttocks, abdominal, and thigh muscles
page 87
6 to 20 times

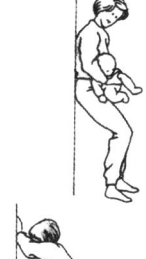

WALL PUSH-UPS
Chest, shoulder, and upper arm muscles
page 88
10 to 20 times

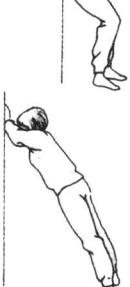

Post workout relaxation
Try lying on your back on the floor (see page 43). Relax like this for at least five minutes.

ENCOURAGING MUSCLE CONTROL

After six weeks a baby's physical development begins to be more noticeable and there are ways you can help enhance this natural progress. Exercises and games with your baby ought to be fun. Remember that they are not a serious activity and should be accompanied by talk and cuddles. Never try them when your baby is hungry, tired, or not feeling well, and stop as soon as the baby starts to cry for any reason. Make sure that he is comfortably dressed and that his clothes do not restrict activities, ideally wearing just a diaper and undershirt if the room is warm and the surface soft. A washable quilt on the floor may be an ideal surface for the exercises, as it is firm, soft, and clean.

By about eight weeks your baby will have begun to focus and be interested in watching a moving toy; he can usually follow it from one side to just beyond the midline. At the same time the reflex that kept his hands tightly fisted as a new baby is disappearing and he is generally less curled and floppy. In the next few weeks these open hands and more relaxed arms are going to begin exploring his clothes and bedding. He is still unable to hold a rattle for more than a few moments, and it is not until after he has begun to lie and play with his own hands (about twelve weeks onward) that he will understand the vital relationship between eyes and hands and begin to reach for what he wants. He shows his excitement at seeing a bright toy held in front of him by kicking and waving his arms furiously and he may hit it by chance but is still unable to explore it.

Helping your baby to play

Although he has not yet learned to grasp an object, he wants very much to do so. Choose objects that are reasonably large, lightweight, and bright, and make a noise when banged, and hang one or two of them over his crib or infant seat; he will swipe at them with his arms and occasionally make contact, perhaps producing a noise that draws his attention to what his hands are doing. A large, fluffy ball with a bell inside, brightly colored teething rings, or an aluminum foil plate can be just as absorbing as an expensive "educational" toy. Once you have engineered the hanging device, perhaps with just a piece of elastic, you can use your ingenuity to think of exciting changes. As long as they are light, have no sharp edges, and are fastened securely, then you have an almost endless supply in your own home.

Visual control

By about twelve to sixteen weeks a baby will have begun to turn his head toward the source of a sound and he can follow a moving object with his eyes from one side over to the other. You can make a game of this activity to help stimulate these vital head and visual movements.

To encourage your baby's visual control, catch his attention so he follows your face with his eyes.

Lay your baby on his back and dangle a bright rattle above him, about 12–16 in (30–40 cm) away, to catch his attention. Slowly move it in an arc, waiting for his eyes and head to follow

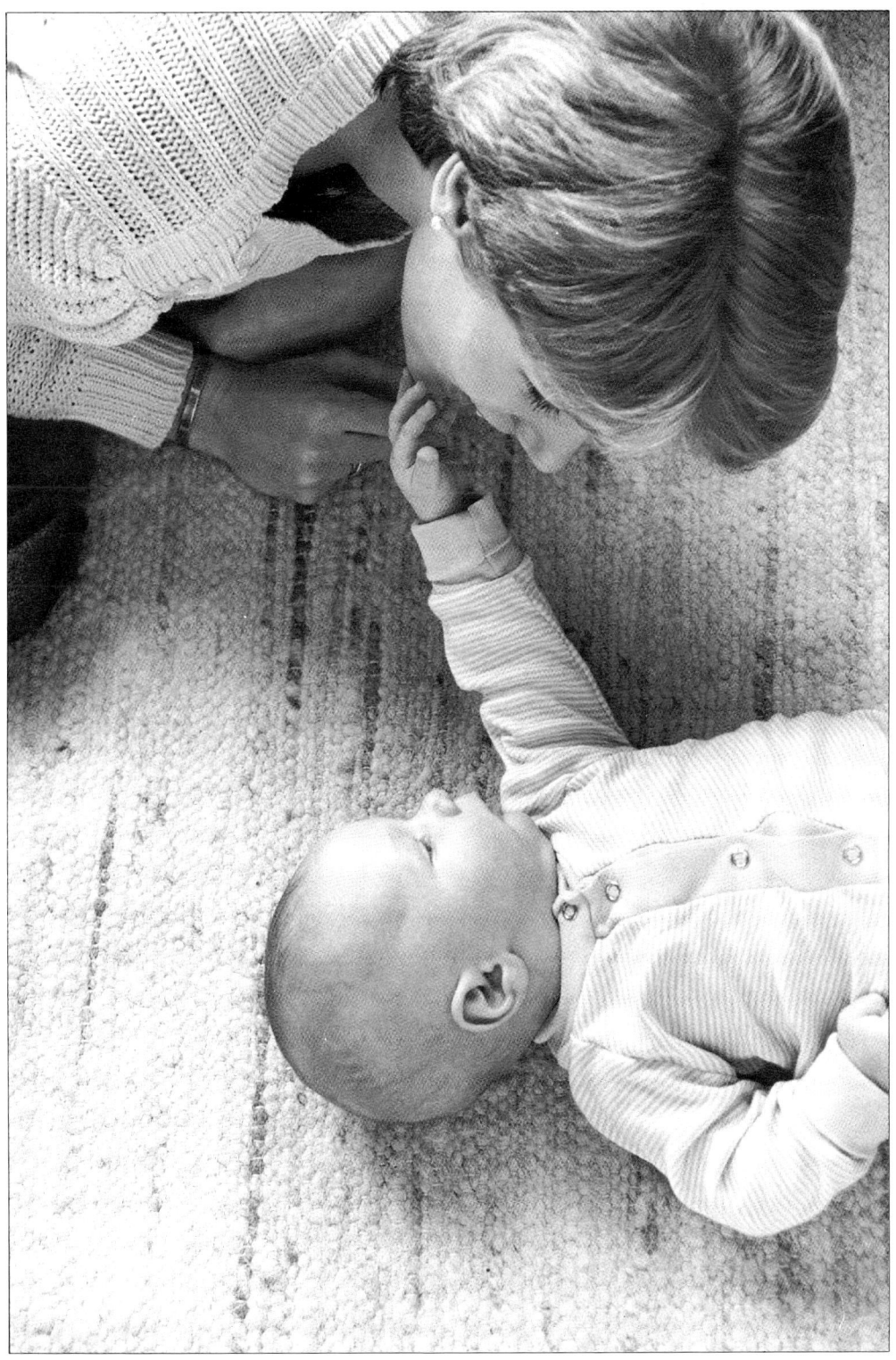

it – rattle it to revive his interest if he loses it. Try moving the rattle back to the midline, and beyond it toward the opposite side as well.

Some babies may cooperate in this game far better if it is a familiar face they are required to follow. Try moving your face from the middle to one side, back to the middle, and over to the opposite side, talking all the time to keep your baby's attention.

Developing head control

Strengthening front neck muscles

Encourage your baby's development of head control by laying him along your thighs and lifting him slowly toward you while you talk to him.

By about two months your baby will be beginning to use his neck muscles to control his head when he is pulled to sitting. You can encourage this important ability by practicing it gently with him when he is seated on your lap.

Sit comfortably with your feet raised on a footstool. Lay your baby lengthwise along your thighs, meanwhile talking to him. Put your thumbs into his palms and wrap your fingers around the back of his hands, turning his palms toward one another. Now straighten his elbows and start to lift his head and body gently toward you, talking to him as you do so. Wait a moment and you will see his head begin to lift in line with his shoulders. Pull him slowly up toward you as far as he can manage while keeping his head controlled and in line with his body, and then lower him gently back. This strengthens his neck muscles and

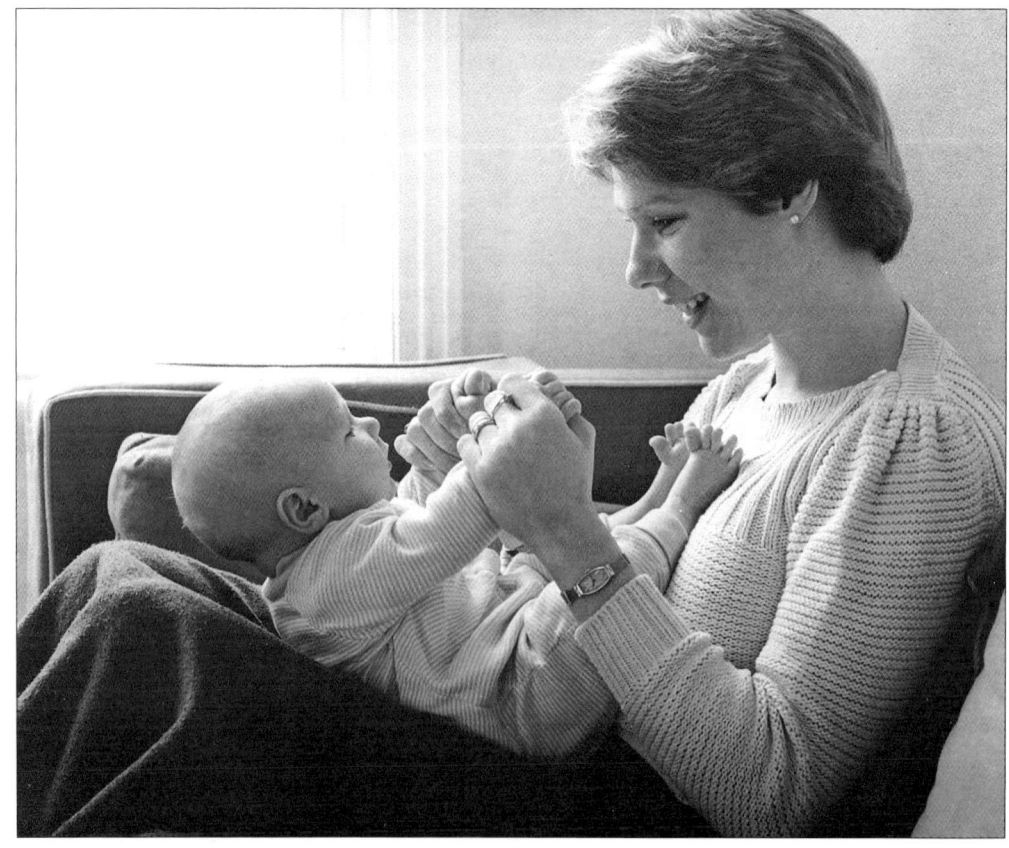

Babies love to be handled, and tipping your baby gently to one side (making sure his head is always in line with his body) makes a delightful game. Do not tilt so far that his head drops down.

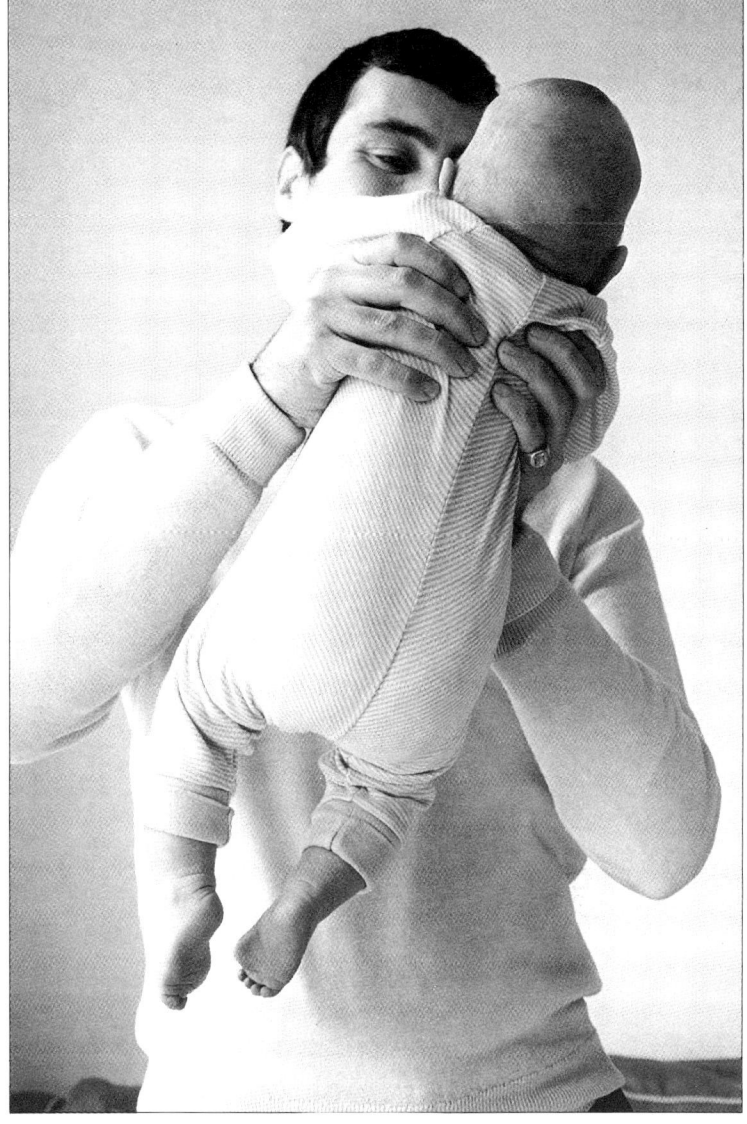

Strengthening side neck muscles

helps him learn to control his head in preparation for sitting.

Another way to stimulate his head control is by tilting him sideways, making sure you allow him time to keep his head in line with his body. Stand with your feet comfortably apart, holding your baby under his arms as you tilt him. Your head and shoulders will tilt also and you can talk to him as he holds this position for a few moments; then slowly return to the middle and tilt him the other way.

By about three months his neck muscles should be able to keep his head steady when he is tilted from side to side. Doing this gently as an exercise will help strengthen these muscles, and your baby will love it, provided he is not tired or hungry.

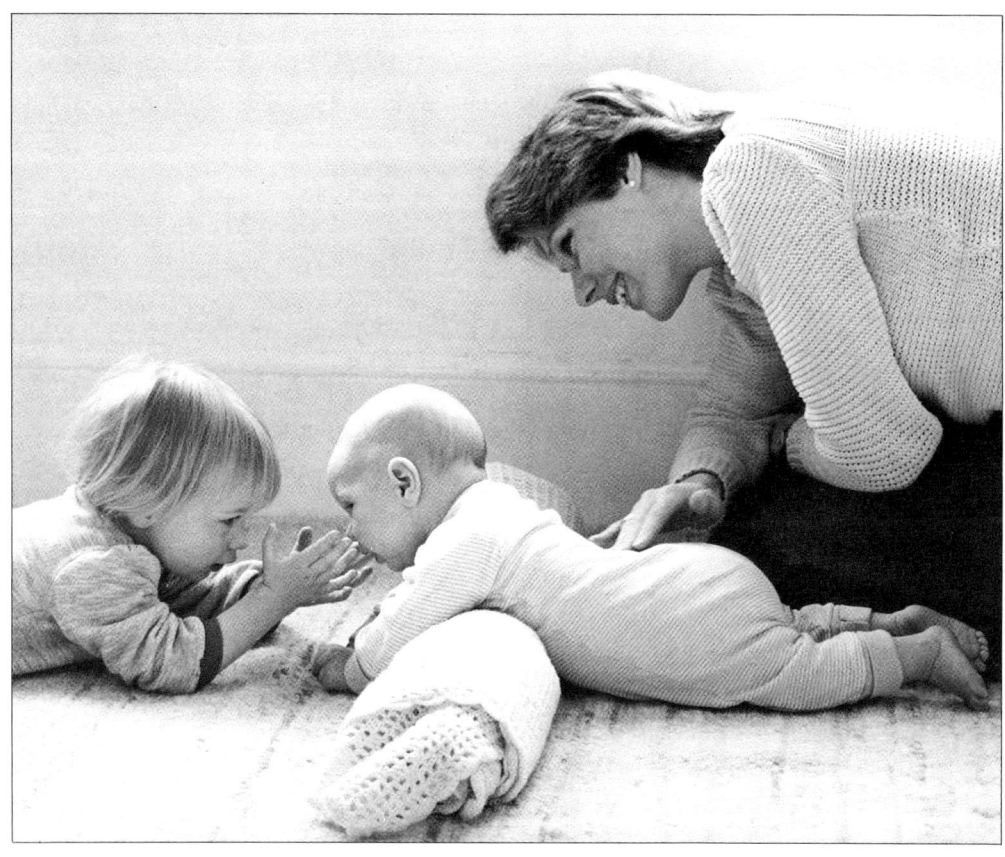

Strengthening your baby's back

It is important for all babies to spend some time lying on their stomachs. Placing a rolled towel under your baby's shoulders helps to strengthen his back, while an elder brother or sister may enjoy being involved as well to attract the baby's attention.

By now your baby is probably needing less sleep during the day, and is no longer happy to be put straight back to bed after every feeding. When you hold him you will notice he is beginning to look around and that he is getting stronger and can lift his chin off the mattress when lying on his stomach.

Help to strengthen your baby's back with the following exercise. Roll up a clean towel to about eight thicknesses – about 2½ in (6 cm) in diameter – and place it on the floor. Gently lower your baby onto his stomach so that his forearms rest on the floor and the towel is under his chest. Now talk to him or use a toy to attract his attention so that he lifts his head up. He will begin to work the muscles of his neck and back – some of the muscles he needs to strengthen for sitting – and learn to take weight through his forearms. You may find that gently rubbing or pressing his spine will help stimulate him to lift his head and straighten his back. Repeat this activity several times a day for as long as your baby is happy. If your baby is not used to lying on his stomach and cries when first put in this position, see if you can distract or soothe him for a few minutes before lifting him up, and try the position again a little later.

Strengthening neck and shoulders

While you are enjoying socializing with your baby, you can also be encouraging him to strengthen the muscles of his neck

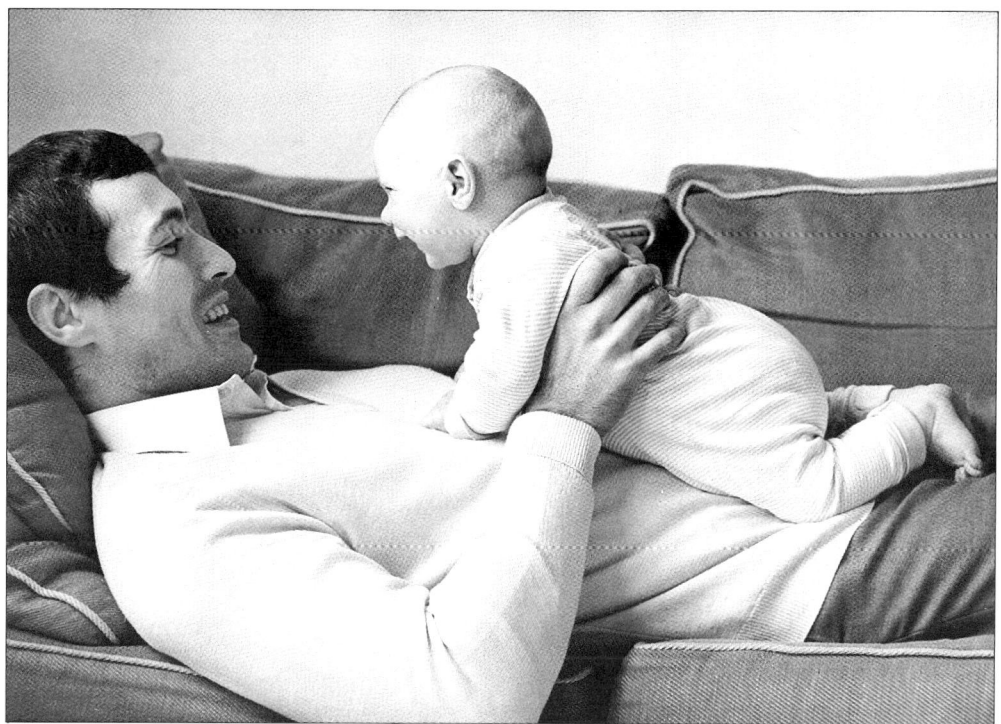

While they enjoy each other's smiles, in this rewarding game father can relax while his baby strengthens his neck, arms, and back.

and shoulders. Lie comfortably on a sofa with your head propped on an armrest and your baby on your chest. Bring his elbows forward and in so that they lie beneath his shoulders and he can support some weight through his forearms. Talk to him so that he wants to lift his head to look at you and, as he does so, you will feel him pressing down through his elbows and forearms and you can lessen your support accordingly. Repeat this wonderfully friendly activity as often and for as long as you both enjoy it.

Using an infant seat

If you haven't already done so, now is the time you may decide to buy your baby her first "chair," an infant seat, made of fabric or firm plastic. She is well supported in an infant seat, and is also tilted slightly upward so that she can watch you while you are busy. You can suspend things of interest in front of her. This type of seat is safe until the baby has started to lift up her head and shoulders, which may be at about five months. While she plays in it, the increasing movements of her arms and legs will gently rock the frame, and that in itself usually delights her even more. It is also light and portable enough for you to take around the house as you move from room to room, but remember that even the smallest rocking motions are enough to move the chair, and it is *never* safe to place it on a table or kitchen counter even for a moment. Frequent changes of position and activity will keep your baby amused during her increasingly long waking hours.

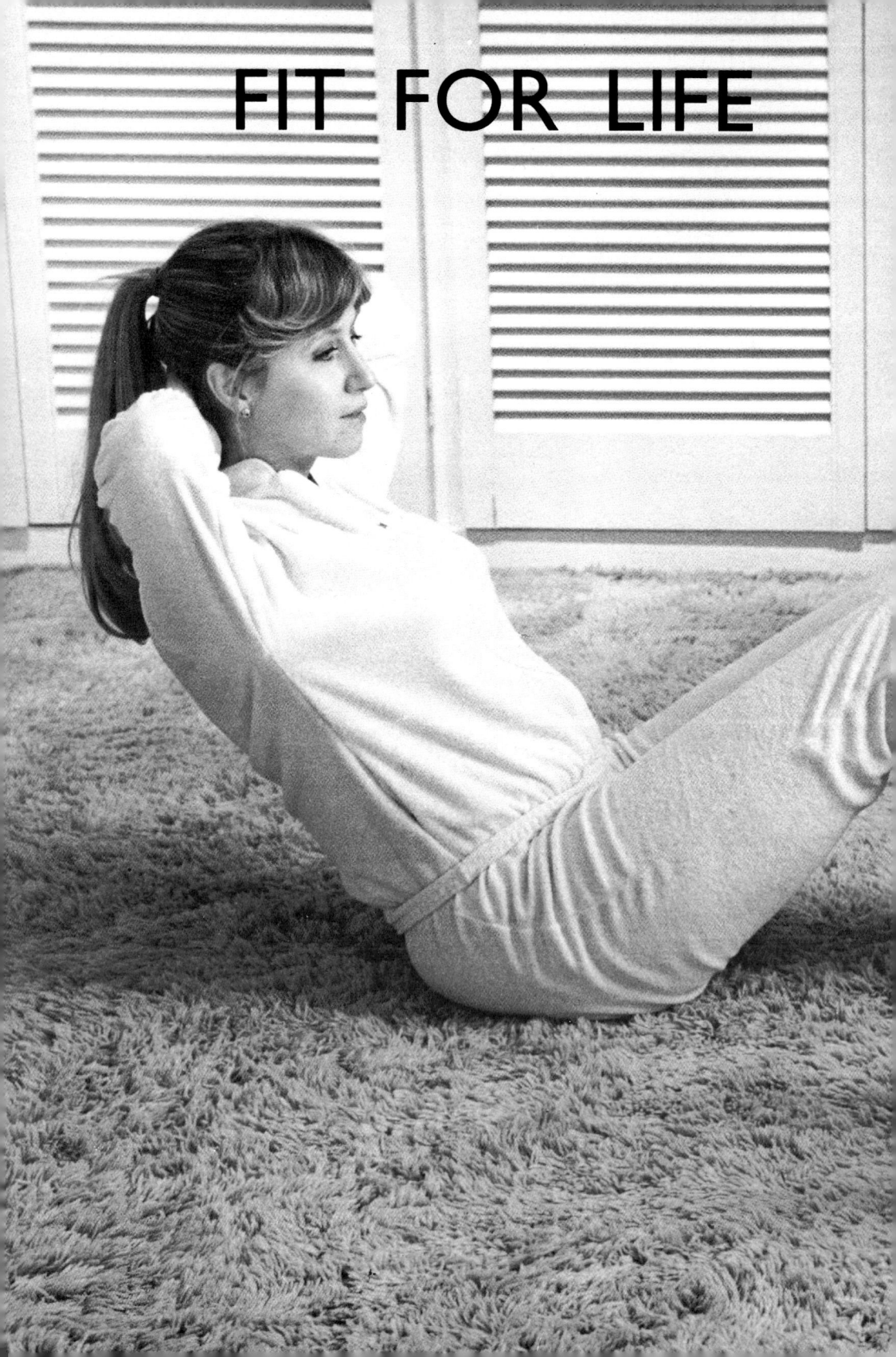
FIT FOR LIFE

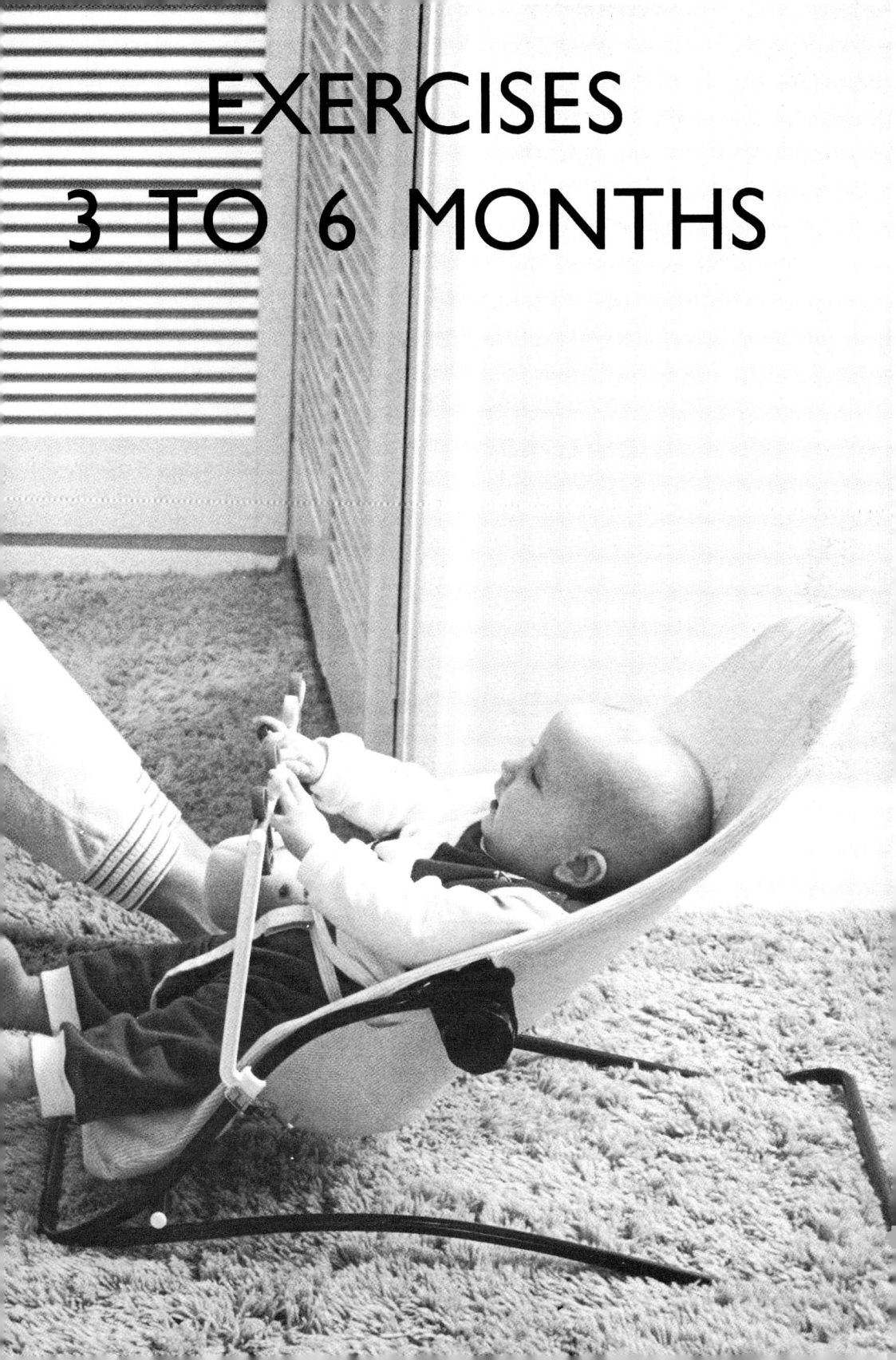

EXERCISES
3 TO 6 MONTHS

If you have been able to do your exercises with some regularity and enthusiasm, your muscles will now be much stronger and firmer and your body will look and feel better than it did. Even if your baby hasn't allowed you time for yourself and you have been unable to do any but the most basic exercises, don't despair. It's never too late to start.

The exercises in this section are very much stronger and will therefore do much more for your figure. If you feel confident about the strength of your muscles, it is perfectly safe to follow the program exactly. However, if you are uncertain, start slowly and gently – keeping the repetitions to a minimum until you are sure that you are not straining yourself. The test given on page 52 to find the gap between the vertical abdominal muscles will tell you what progress you have made. By now you should find that the gap has nearly closed and that your muscles feel much firmer. Remember that it is normal for a tiny gap to persist above and below your umbilicus, and for the space to be somewhat larger at umbilical level. The torn strip of fibrous tissue (page 19) does not regenerate, but the strength and function of the abdominal muscles are not affected. Opposite you will find a strenuous test for that other group of important muscles – the pelvic floor.

If excess weight is still a problem, watch your diet; cookies, cakes, candy, potato chips, nuts, and other snacks are very high in calories and not essential in a well-balanced eating plan. To help burn up fat it is necessary to exercise at moderate intensity for more than twenty minutes at a time at least four to five times each week. Even if you feel too tired, it is worth making an effort because many people find aerobic exercise gives an emotional as well as a physical "lift."

Your baby by now will be quite delightful and thoroughly rewarding. Apart from allowing her to join you in your exercises, you will want to use your playtimes with her to help her physical progress in every way. She is rapidly learning to control her head, limbs, and body and you will find that very soon she will be rolling and sitting. She will already be communicating her needs and pleasures very clearly and using her voice in various ways. Exercising with her now should be great fun for you both.

Soon you will want to move on from the restricting, and sometimes solitary, routine of postnatal exercises and will be wondering when it is safe to resume a normal sport, exercise, or dance class. Obviously this will depend enormously on how fit you were just before your baby's birth, and the type of sport you are planning to take up. In the section "Resuming Normal Exercise" (page 123) there is some basic advice on your choices and the activities that are still best avoided. By the time your baby is six months old you should certainly feel "Fit for Life!"

PELVIC FLOOR MUSCLE STRENGTHENING

THE ULTIMATE TEST

By the time your baby is six months old you should no longer have any discomfort from your stitches and the strength of your pelvic floor muscles should be enough to control your bladder when you cough, sneeze, or pick up your baby.

The ultimate test for your pelvic floor control is to jump up and down on the spot, eventually trying with your legs apart, coughing at the same time – your underpants should stay dry. This does not mean that you can forget your pelvic floor exercises until you have your next baby. Ideally, every woman should be aware at all times of this hammock of muscles and the role it plays in her day to day activities and sex life, so continue tightening, and holding hard for six to eight seconds, then relaxing these muscles a few times a day for the rest of your life. It is also a good idea to get into the habit of bracing your pelvic muscles whenever you cough, sneeze, or lift anything heavy.

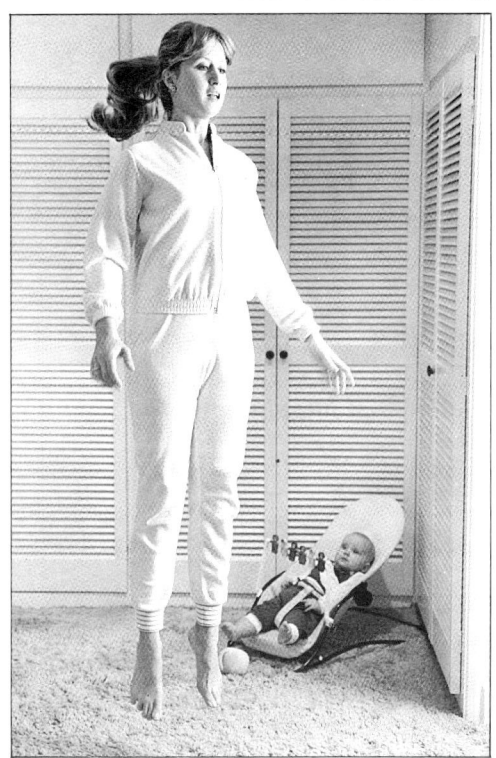

DEEP KNEE SQUATS

Squat down, preferably with your heels flat on the floor, holding onto a chair if you find it difficult to balance yourself. If you can't keep your heels down comfortably, squat on your toes with your heels raised, or try it with shoes on (a small heel sometimes makes all the difference). Your pelvic floor muscles have to work harder in this position than when you are sitting, standing, or lying.

Tighten the ring of muscles around your anus, and draw the vaginal muscles inward and upward; at the same time, try and feel the contraction of the muscles around your front passage (urethra) too. Hold this squeeze for eight seconds, increasing the power of your contraction for the last three (see page 75). Repeat ten times. Remember you can do this exercise in any position.

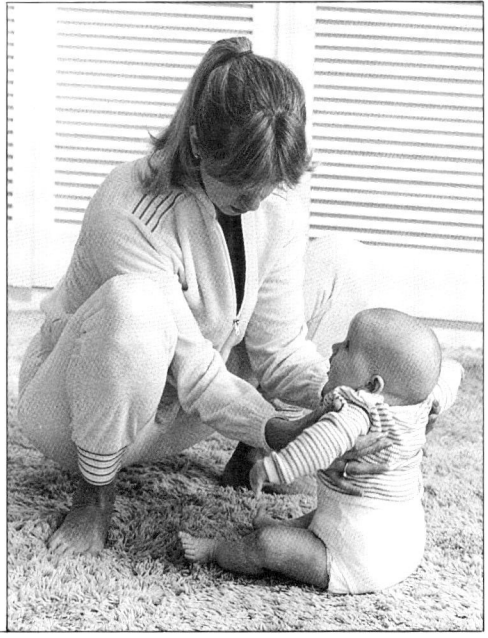

LYING ON THE FLOOR

PELVIC THRUSTS

This exercise is good for your pelvic floor, buttock, and back muscles.

Lie on the floor with your heels resting on a low chair or box. Your baby can lie or sit on your stomach. Tighten your pelvic floor muscles, drawing inward and upward; at the same time squeeze your buttocks tightly together and raise your bottom off the floor so that your body is in a straight line from your heels to your head. Hold this position for four counts and then lower. Do it six times and increase to twelve. This exercise can be progressed by holding your bottom in the air for longer – up to ten counts.

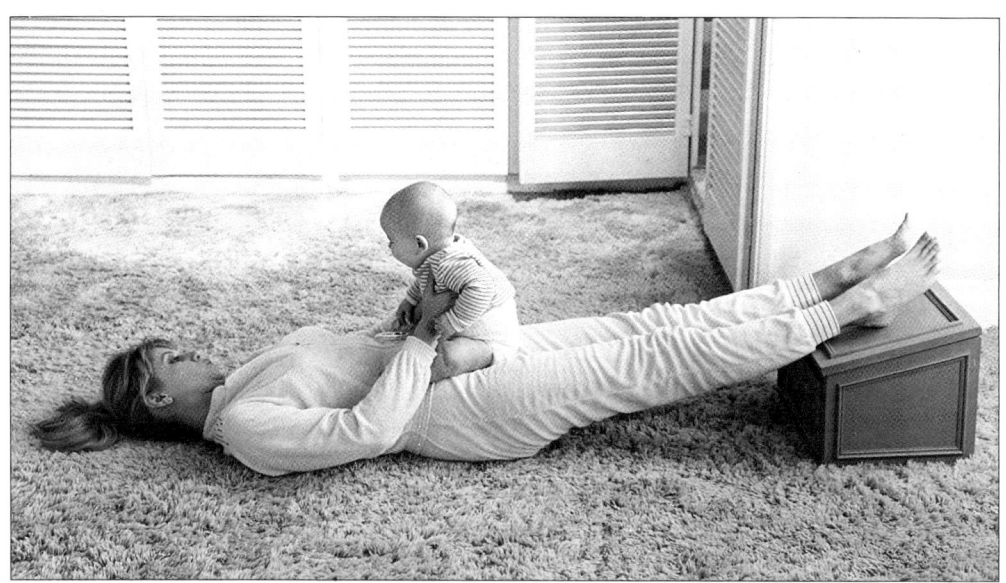

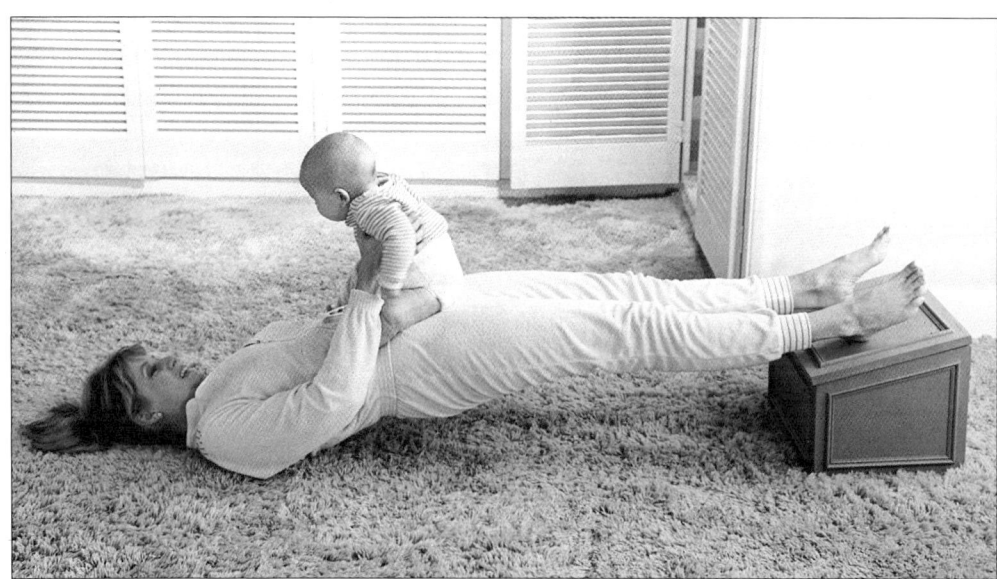

CYCLING

This exercise is good for your leg and abdominal muscles.

Lie on your back with your knees bent up to your chest. Blow out, draw your abdominal muscles in, and lift your head from the floor. Keeping your left knee pulled up close to you, stretch the right leg out until it is straight and 6 in (15 cm) from the floor. With a cycling motion, change legs so that your left leg is then stretched out. Repeat for six sequences, then bend both knees and lower your feet to the floor. Progress to twenty sequences.

It is vital that you brace your abdominal muscles and make sure that your waist is pressed down firmly on the floor throughout the movement. If your back is arching up as you "cycle" your legs, it indicates that you are not yet ready for this strong exercise. Concentrate on the less strenuous ones for now.

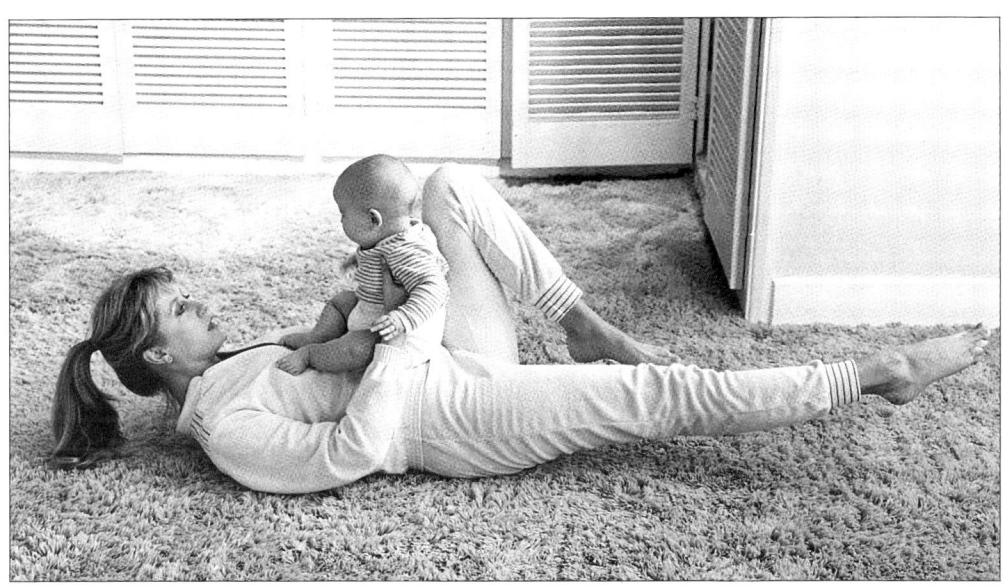

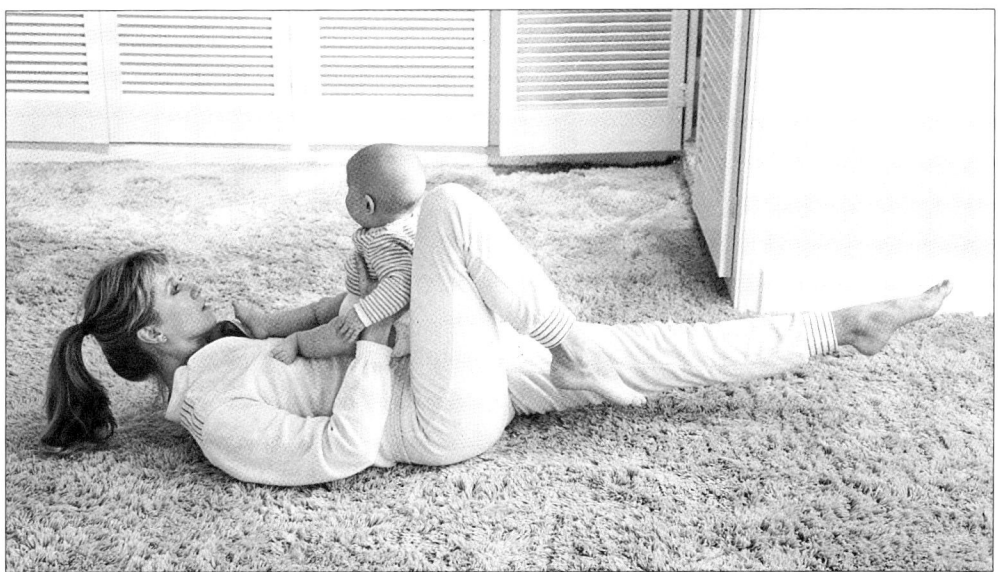

LATERAL FLEXED KNEE TWISTS

This exercise slims the waist and hips.

Lie on your back with your hands behind your head and your legs straight. Holding your knees and feet together, blow out, pull in your stomach, and bend your knees up tightly onto your chest. Keeping your abdominal muscles pulled well in, let your knees roll slowly to the right until your thigh touches the floor, making sure that both elbows are still pressed down hard. Rest for a moment; then, pulling in your abdominal muscles once again, bring your knees up to the middle. Repeat to the left. Do this sequence six times and increase to twenty-four.

This exercise can be progressed by moving the knees from side to side without pausing in the middle, and also by increasing the speed of the movement.

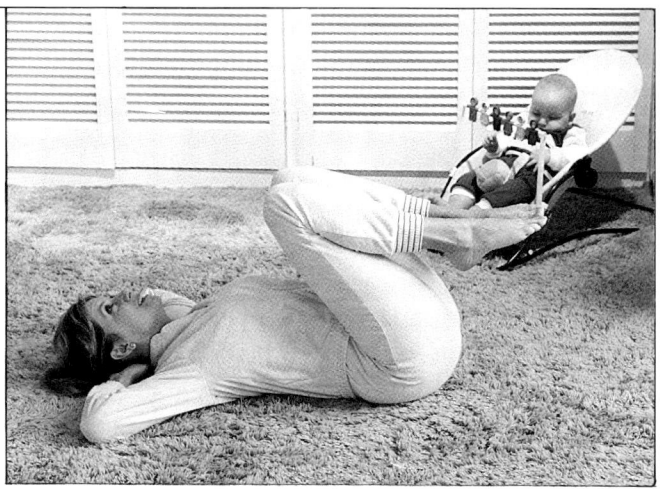

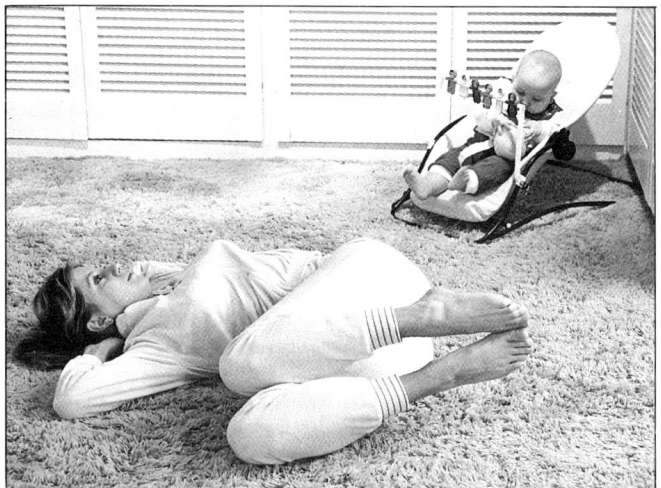

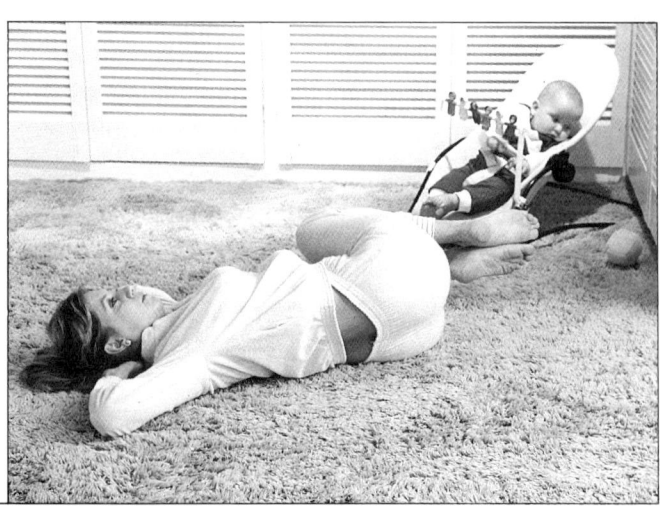

SCISSORS

This exercise tones, shapes, and strengthens your thighs and also your abdominal muscles.

Lie on your back with your legs straight. Blow out, pull in your stomach muscles, and bend both legs together onto your chest, keeping your back pressed to the floor. If you are unable to do this yet, slide both feet up to your buttocks and then bend your knees up onto your chest. Now stretch your legs up so that they are at a right angle to your body. Make sure that you keep your back firmly pressed to the floor throughout this movement. Pulling your abdomen in all the time, open and close your legs, stretching them as wide apart as you can and crossing them first one way and then the other in the middle, like scissors.

Do this eight times, then bend your knees onto your chest and lower your feet back to the floor, still keeping your back pressed down hard. To make this exercise a little more difficult lift your head. Do this sequence four times to start with, progressing to twelve.

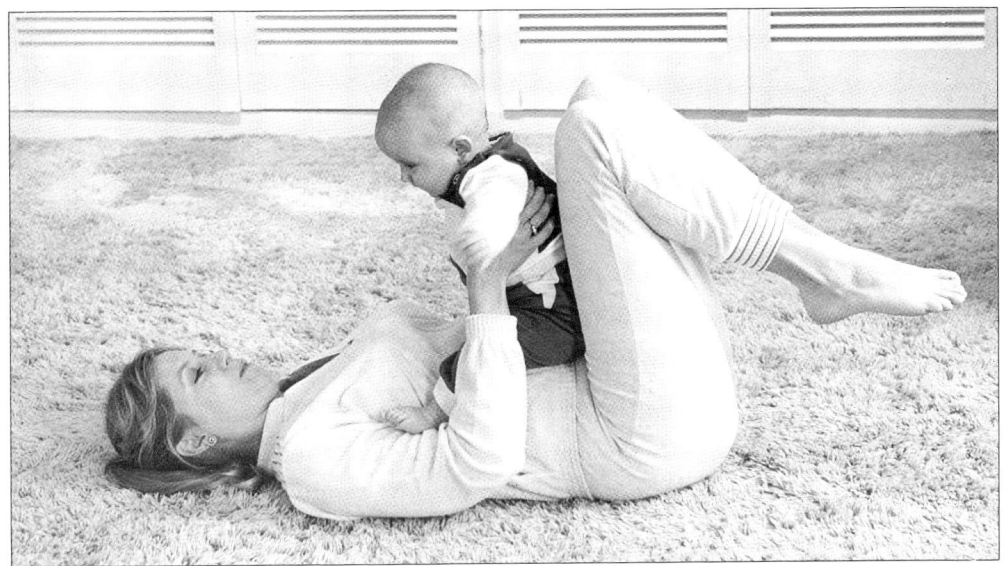

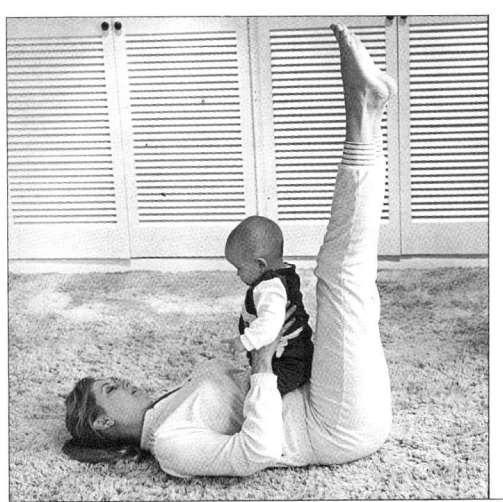
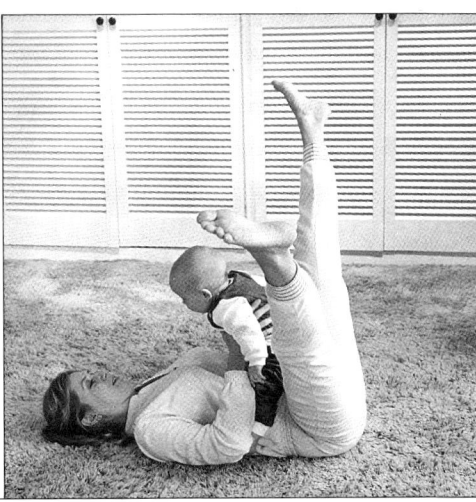

DUAL LEG ABDUCTIONS

This exercise strengthens abdominal and thigh muscles, and helps to trim a thick waist.

Lie on your side, resting your head on your hand, and balancing yourself with your other hand in front of your body.

Tuck in your stomach and buttocks. Blow out, and lift both legs up sideways; hold for four counts and then lower slowly. Do this six times and then turn onto your other side and repeat. Start with six leg lifts; then progress by increasing to twelve each side.

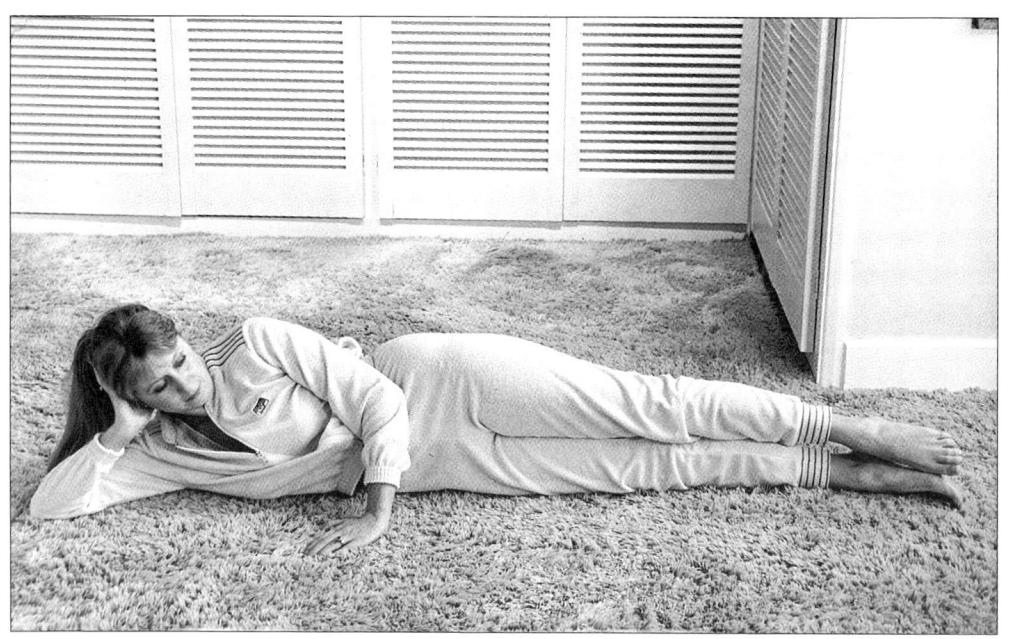

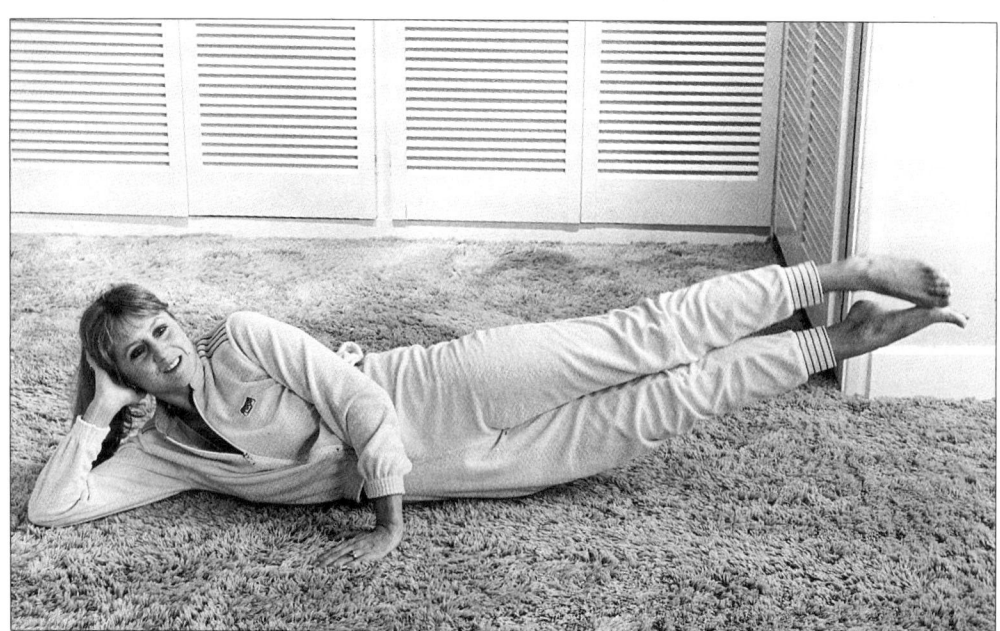

SITTING ON THE FLOOR

FULL SIT-UPS

This exercise will continue strengthening and tightening your straight abdominal muscles, returning them to full normality.

Sit with your knees bent up high and both arms stretched out in front of you. Blow out, pull in your abdominal muscles, and tuck your buttocks under; then slowly curl downward, allowing your back to reach the floor, vertebra by vertebra. Relax. Blow out and pull your abdominal muscles in again, then curl upward so that you are sitting up straight once more. This exercise can be progressed by omitting the relaxing pause when you reach the floor and then by putting your hands behind your head.

Only begin this very strong exercise when you feel you can really control the movement without collapsing back onto the floor or having to jerk yourself up to begin the sit-up. Start with four and progress to sixteen.

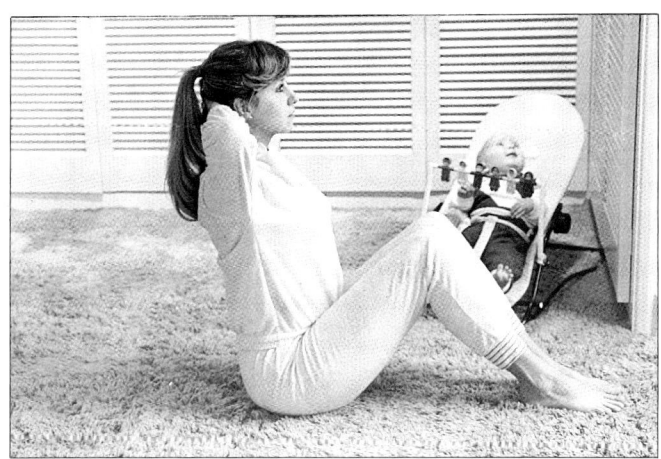

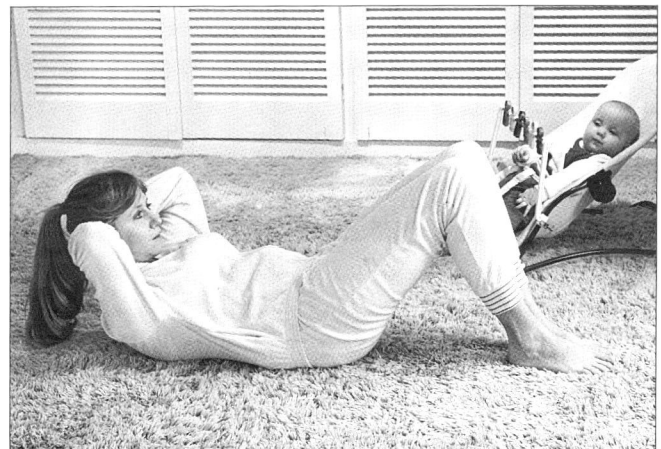

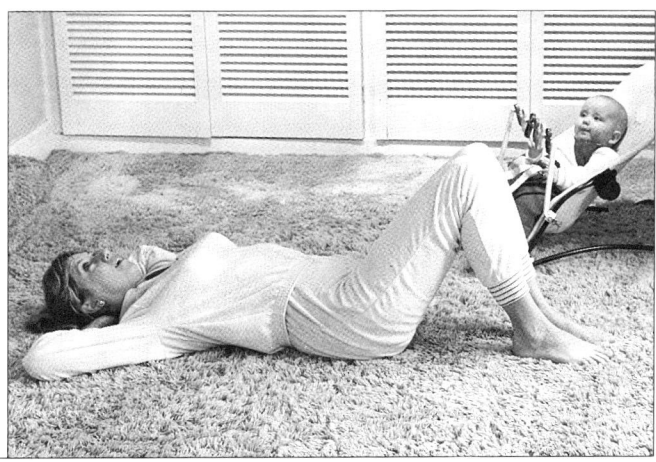

KNEELING EXERCISES

KNEELING TWISTS

This firms your thighs, buttocks, waist, and pelvic floor.

Kneel on the floor with your arms crossed and lifted in front of you or holding your baby as shown. Remembering to keep your abdominal and buttock muscles firmly pulled in, sit yourself on the floor on your right. Now lift up, holding abdomen and buttocks firmly and adding a pelvic floor "lift" at the same time, then change to sitting on your left.

Keep the movement controlled, and don't bump your bottom down too hard on the floor – you will not be working the muscles effectively and you may bruise yourself. Start with eight, then progress to sixteen and finally to twenty-four.

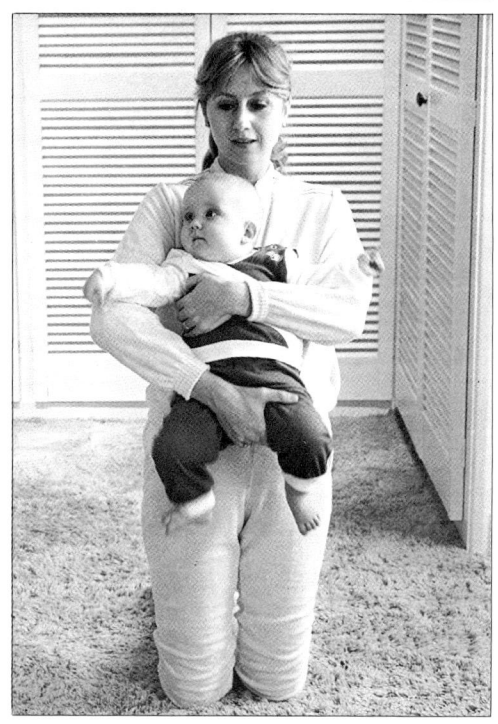

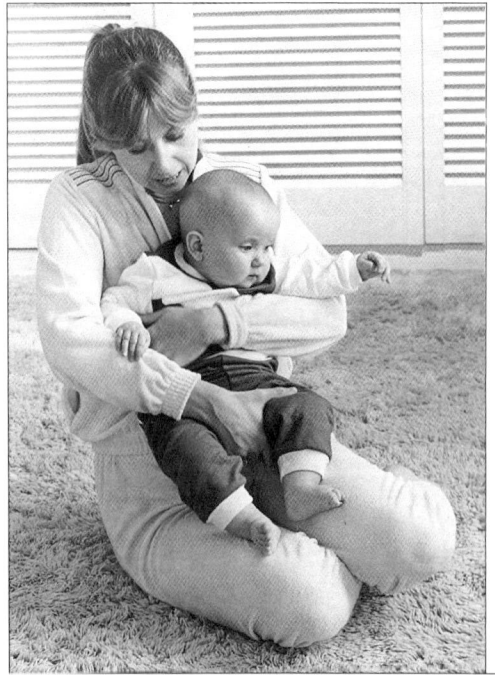

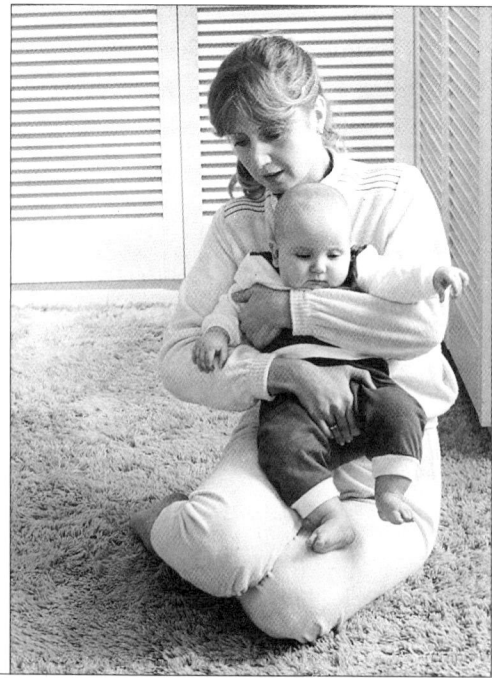

LEANBACKS

This exercise will firm your thighs, buttocks, abdominal muscles, and pelvic floor.

Kneel with both arms stretched out in front of you. Tuck your bottom under, your stomach in, and lift your pelvic floor up, blow out and lean back slowly as far as you can. Hold the position for four counts and then return to your starting position. Start with six leanbacks and increase to twenty. You can make this exercise harder by holding your baby in your arms in front of you. Do it in front of a mirror so that your baby will be amused to see you both come and go as you lean back and straighten up (see pages 117–8).

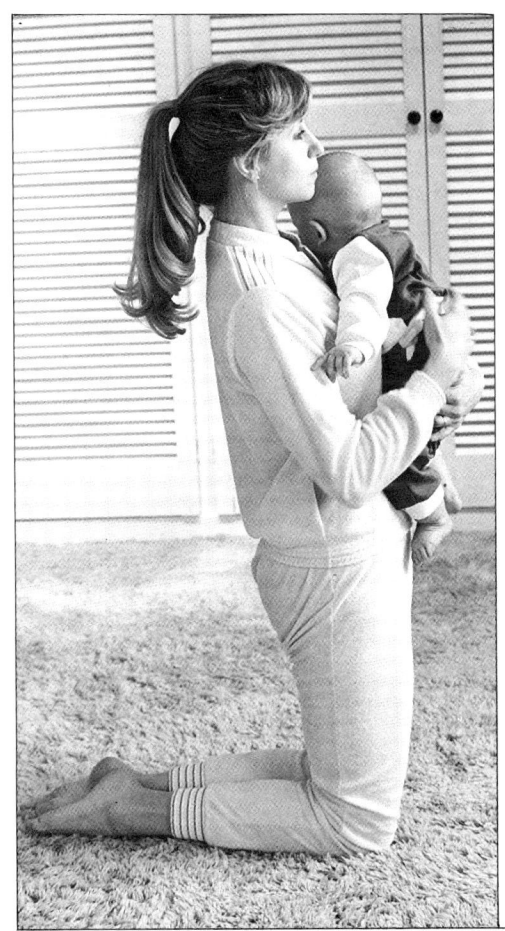
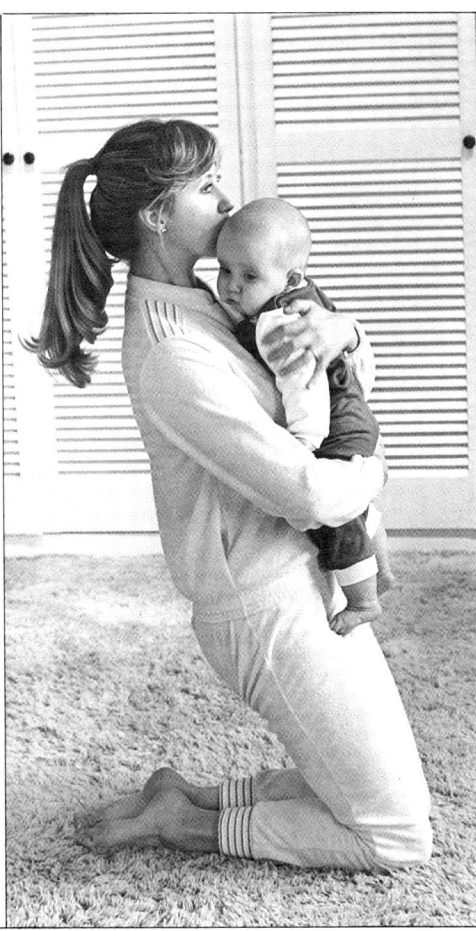

THE FINAL TEST

ELBOW TO KNEE LATERAL SIT-UPS

This exercise makes all your abdominal muscles work very powerfully, testing the work you have been putting into them.

Lie on your back with both knees bent up high and your hands behind your head. Pull in your abdominal muscles firmly, blow out, and tuck your chin onto your chest, bringing your left elbow to touch your right knee. Hold for four counts and lower slowly. Repeat to the other side using the opposite elbow and knee. This exercise can be made harder by holding the elbow-to-knee position longer, and then by keeping both feet flat on the floor as you come up.

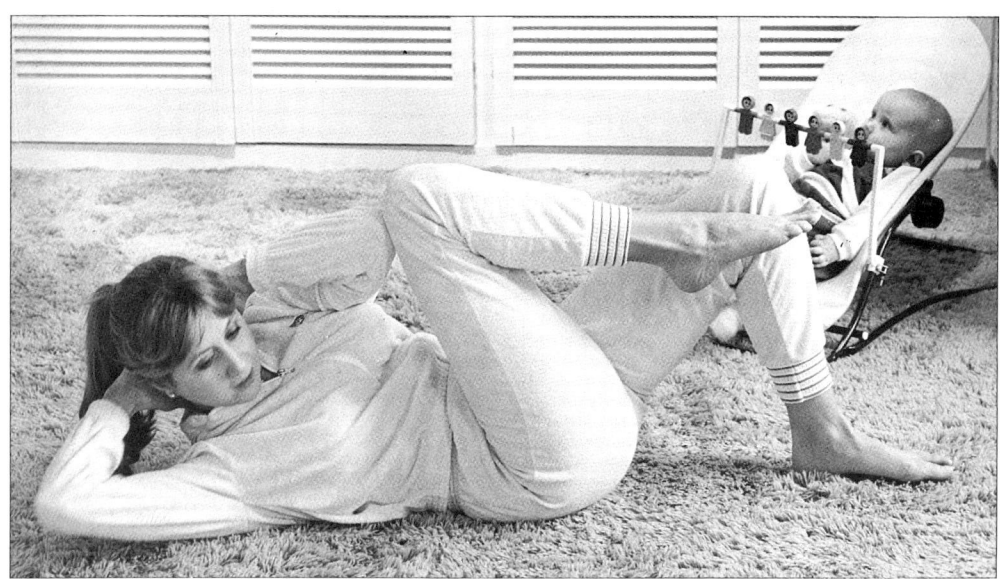

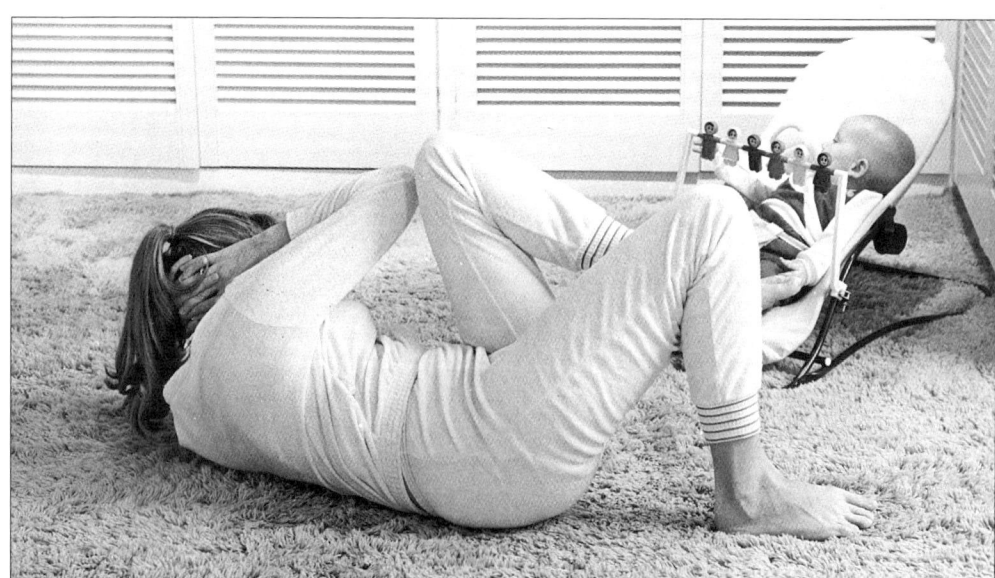

AT THE SWIMMING POOL

LATERAL KNEE RAISES

This exercise works the vertical abdominal muscles as you draw your knees to your chest and the diagonal (oblique) abdominal muscles as you twist, trimming your waist.

Stand with your back to the sides of the pool, stretching your arms out along the rail. Pull in your abdominal muscles, and draw your knees up to your chest. Hold the position, keeping your knees pressed together and your abdominal muscles tight, while you twist your knees to the right side as far as you can. Hold while you count to four, return to the middle, and repeat the twisting movement to the left. Now return to the middle and relax. Repeat this complete sequence ten times, increasing to twenty.

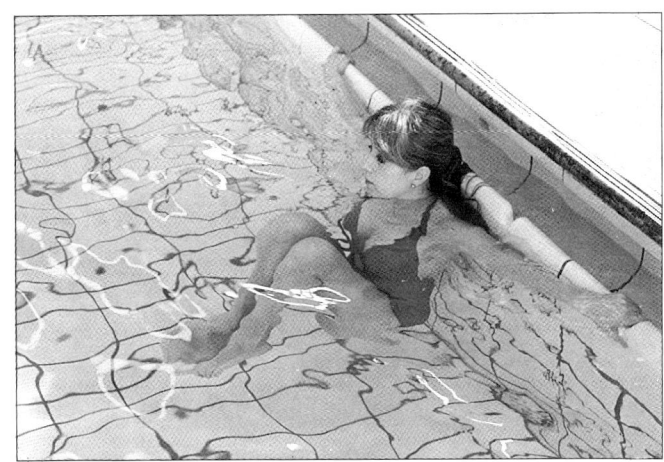

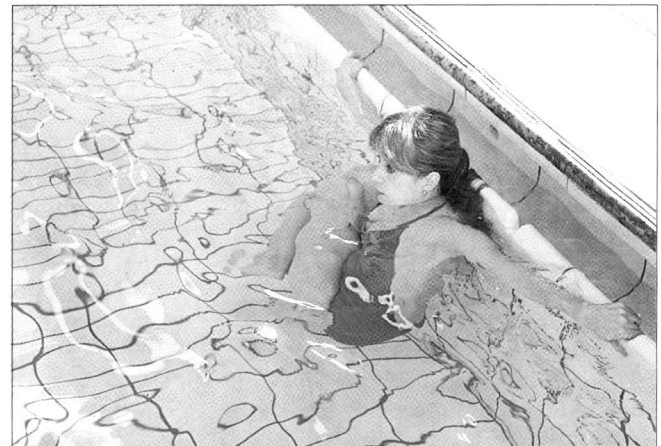

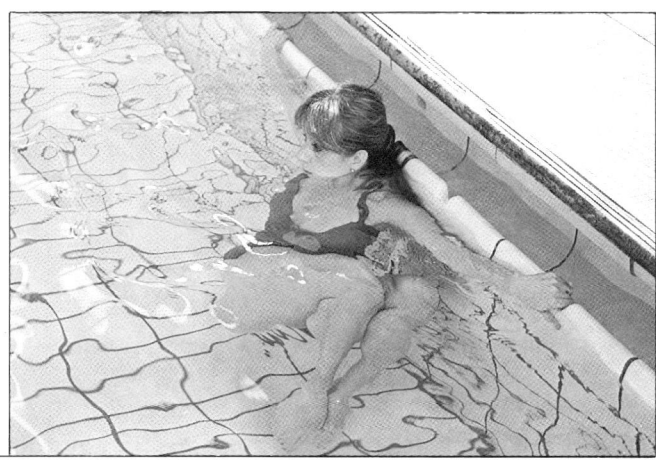

WATER CURL-UPS

This exercise will require your vertical abdominal muscles to work hard against the water's resistance. You will also work your back and buttock muscles to regain and maintain your floating position.

Face the rail at the deep end and hold it with your arms bent and your legs stretched out behind you, so that you are floating. Pull in your abdominal muscles, grip your legs together, and slowly bend your knees up toward your chest. Hold to the count of four, then relax your legs so that they drop down. Now gently kick your legs so that they are once again floating out behind you, and repeat the exercise. Start with ten and increase to twenty times.

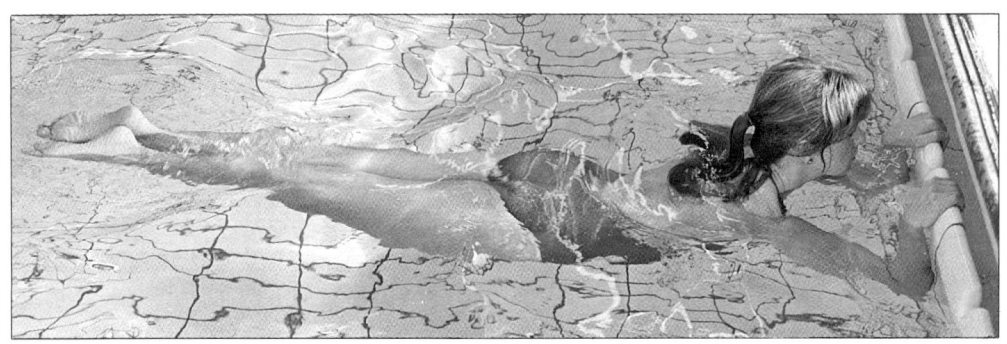

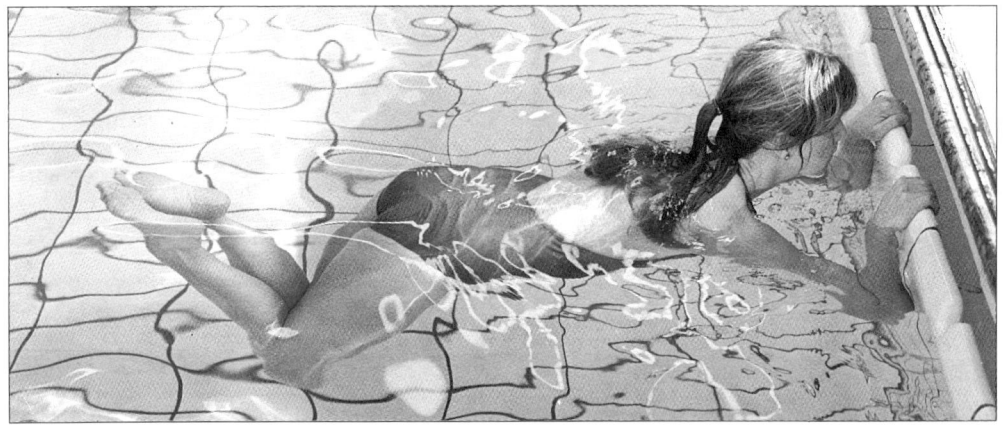

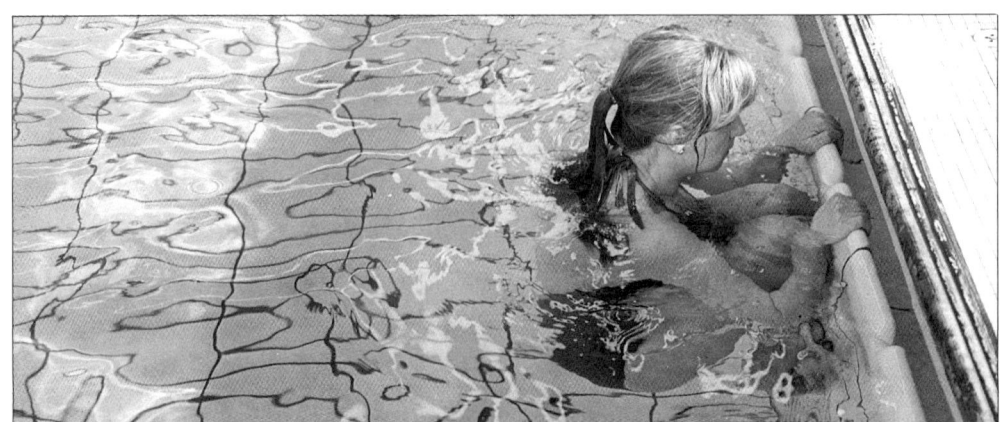

WAIST SWINGS

In this exercise, you are working the muscles at the front and sides of your waist against resistance, firming and strengthening them. At the deep end, hold onto the rail with your back to the side of the pool. Let yourself relax with your legs straight and together, then pull in your abdominal muscles and gently swing your body and legs from the waist down – first to the left, keeping your shoulders and upper trunk still, and then to the right. Repeat ten times to each side, increasing to twenty.

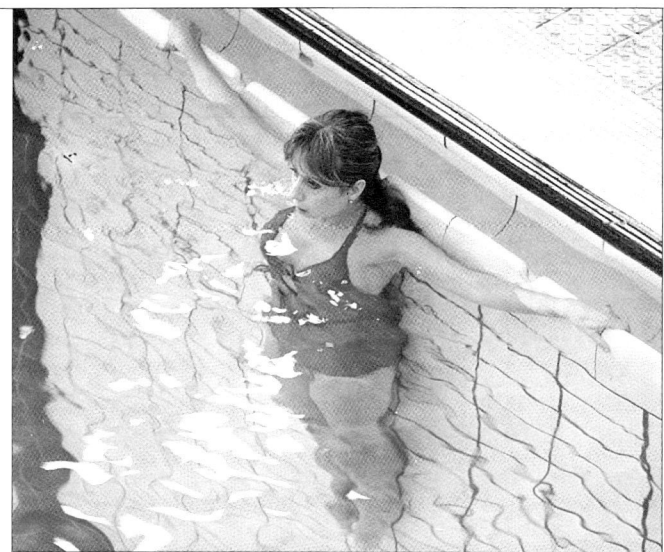

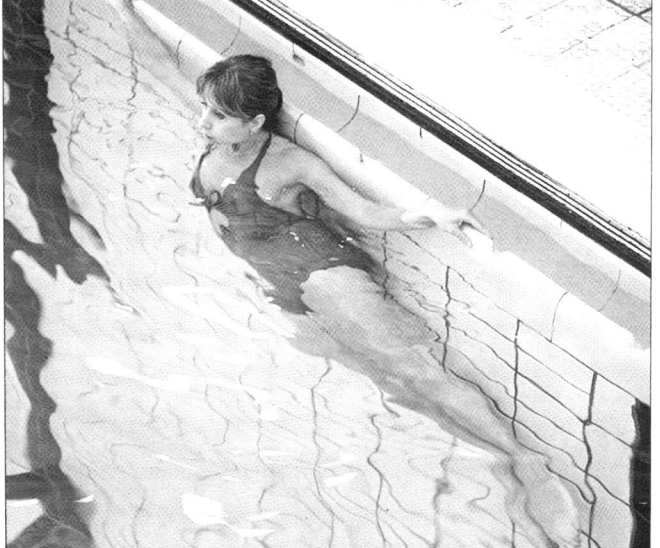

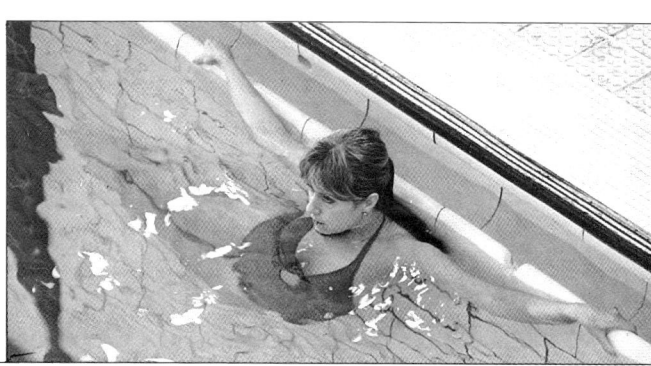

DAILY PROGRAM

Reminder Try to do these exercises the recommended number of times, twice a day. Asterisks mark the most important exercises, so on days when you have very little time at least try to do these.

Pelvic floor muscle strengthening

*DEEP KNEE SQUATS
Pelvic floor muscles
page 99
12 times

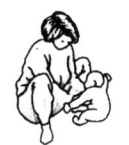

Lying on the floor

PELVIC THRUSTS
Pelvic floor, buttock, and back muscles page 100
6 to 20 times

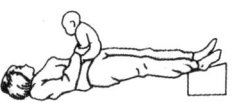

CYCLING
Leg and abdominal muscles
page 101
6 to 20 times

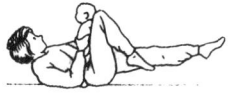

LATERAL FLEXED KNEE TWISTS
Oblique abdominal and lower back muscles
page 102
6 to 20 times

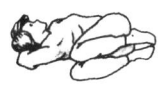

SCISSORS
Thighs and abdominal muscles page 103
4 to 12 times

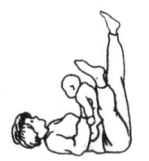

*DUAL LEG ABDUCTIONS
Abdominal and thigh muscles
page 104
4 to 12 times

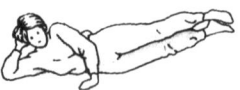

Sitting on the floor

*FULL SIT-UPS
Vertical abdominal muscles page 105
4 to 20 times

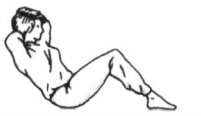

Kneeling exercises

KNEELING TWISTS
Thighs, buttocks, abdominal muscles, and pelvic floor muscles page 106
8 to 20 times

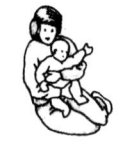

LEANBACKS
Thighs, buttocks, abdominal muscles, and pelvic floor muscles page 107
6 to 20 times

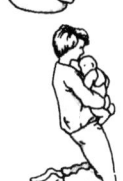

At the swimming pool

LATERAL KNEE RAISES
Vertical and oblique abdominal muscles
page 109 10 to 20 times

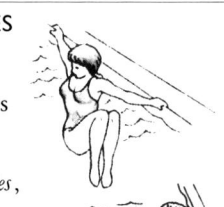

WATER CURL-UPS
Vertical abdominal muscles, back and buttock muscles
page 110
10 to 20 times

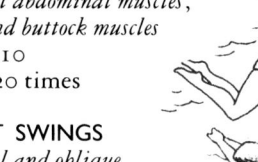

WAIST SWINGS
Vertical and oblique abdominal muscles
page 111 10 to 12 times

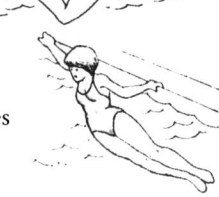

The final tests

When you can do both these exercises you're ready for anything.

*ELBOW TO KNEE LATERAL SIT-UPS
All abdominal muscles
page 108 6 to 20 times

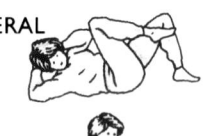

THE ULTIMATE PELVIC FLOOR TEST
Pelvic floor muscles page 99
Do once after the first 3 months and occasionally thereafter

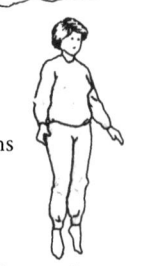

Post workout relaxation
Try lying flat on your back with your legs raised (see page 43). Relax like this for at least five minutes.

LEARNING THROUGH PLAY

For babies, the age of three to six months is an intense period of socializing – they are obviously beginning to understand their surroundings, and are just as capable of excitement at the sight of people or toys they like as they are of anger at being denied something they want. Their heads can now move independently but they do not have full control until about five to six months. Although by four months babies can hold their heads up well while sitting, when they are pulled from a lying position their heads still lag behind at the beginning of the movement.

Helping head control

You can help strengthen your baby's neck muscles by practicing this exercise every time you pick her up from lying down, provided she is not tired or unhappy. Lay your baby on the carpet and kneel down facing her, with one of your knees positioned between her legs. Move your face close to her and catch her attention by talking to her. Put your thumbs in her palms and wrap your fingers around her hands, then gently pull her arms straight and begin to lift her upward. Wait for her to cooperate and work her neck, arm, and stomach muscles – you will see her head begin to pull into line with her body and feel her arm and stomach muscles helping you pull her up. Reward her with a smile or a cuddle each time she does it.

Propped sitting

Another way of helping develop head control is to prop your baby in a sitting position. By three to four months babies

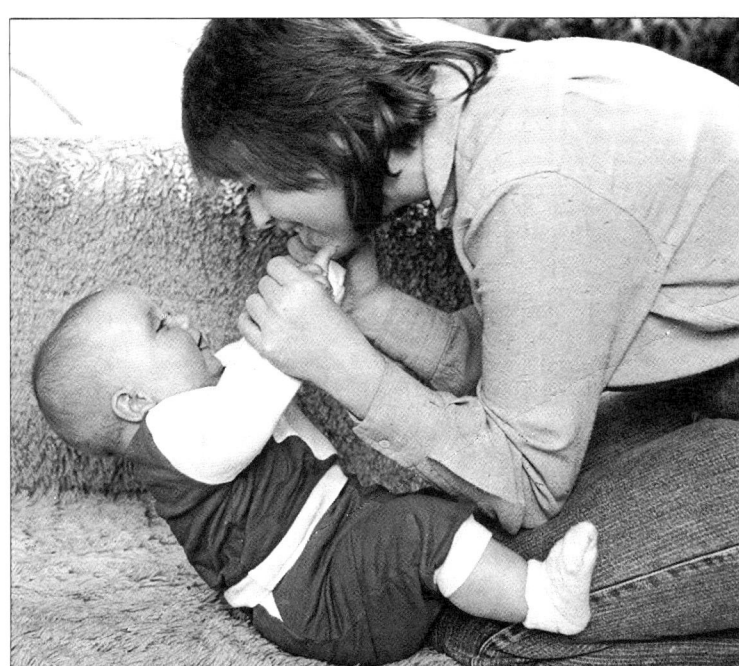

Once your baby is three months old, with supervision an older child – like this baby's sister – can help to develop your baby's vital head control in preparation for sitting.

Right: As early as three to four months, you can prop your baby in a carriage, lessening the support as her strength and control improve. Even at this stage, however, make sure your baby wears a safety harness.
Opposite: Rolling is your baby's first step to mobility. Start by attracting her attention to one side (top), then encourage her to turn by easing her leg over (below), making sure she does most of the work.

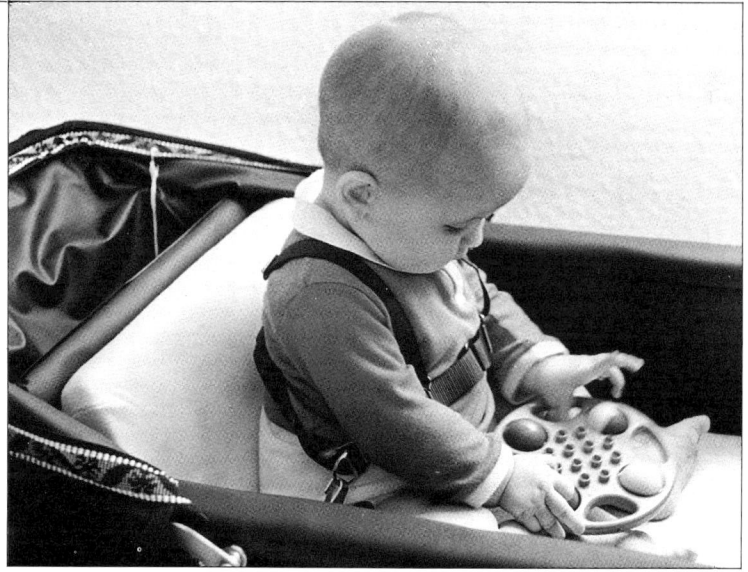

can hold their heads up well enough to enjoy sitting and looking around, their backs being fairly straight, though not yet in the lower part. By five months their heads are even more stable and spines still straighter, and they almost demand to be sat up to watch and play.

A baby carriage is the ideal place to teach your baby the early skills needed for sitting. Use small cushions or folded blankets to prop behind and to the sides as necessary, and a rolled blanket under her thighs if her bottom slips forward. As her sitting improves, move her further upright and lessen her support, but always harness even a young baby for safety. Loosely suspend some rattles on elastic across the carriage so that she can reach for them, but make sure that if she slides down, the elastic will not harm her.

Learning to roll

While your baby is learning how to remain erect in preparation for sitting, she is also beginning to learn to twist or rotate her trunk so that she can roll. (This movement of the body is necessary for crawling, and later, walking, when the leg of one side will move with the arm of the other.) By about five to six months most babies will have learned to roll from their stomachs onto their backs, and by about a month later will be able to roll the other way. You can help your baby roll from an early age when you are changing her diaper – only be careful that you never leave her unattended on a high surface in case she decides she can do it by herself.

Start with your baby on her back, lying on an unrestricted, firm, but comfortable area, for instance, a clean carpet or a blanket on the floor. With your left hand, attract her attention with a bright, noisy rattle about 12 in (30 cm) to the right of her face so that she turns to look at it. Now put your right

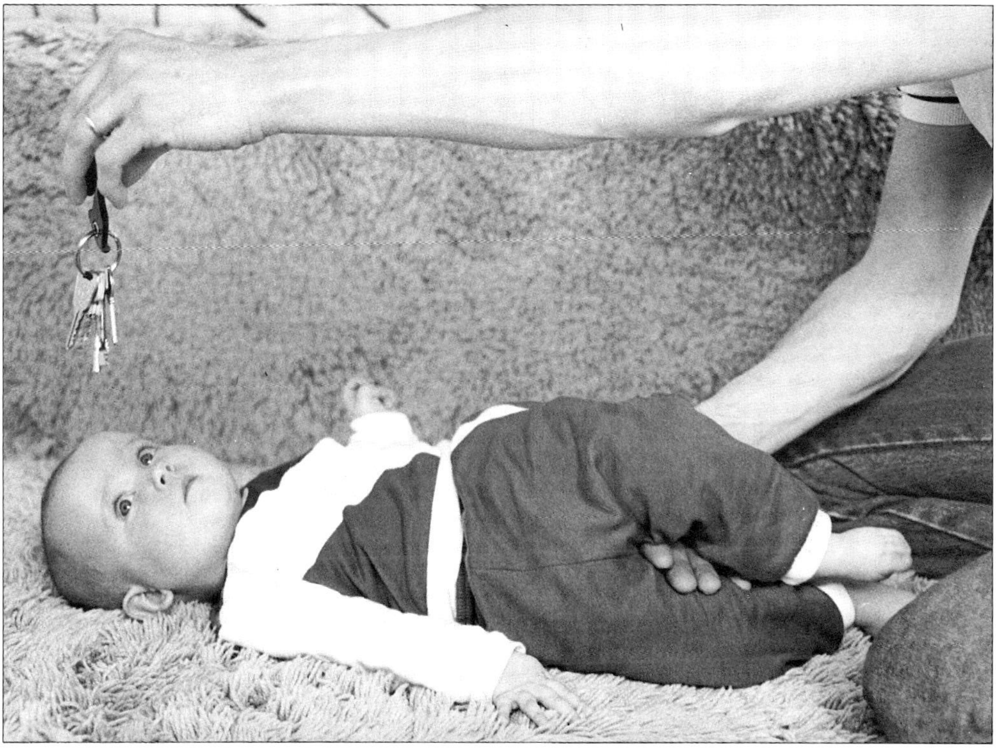

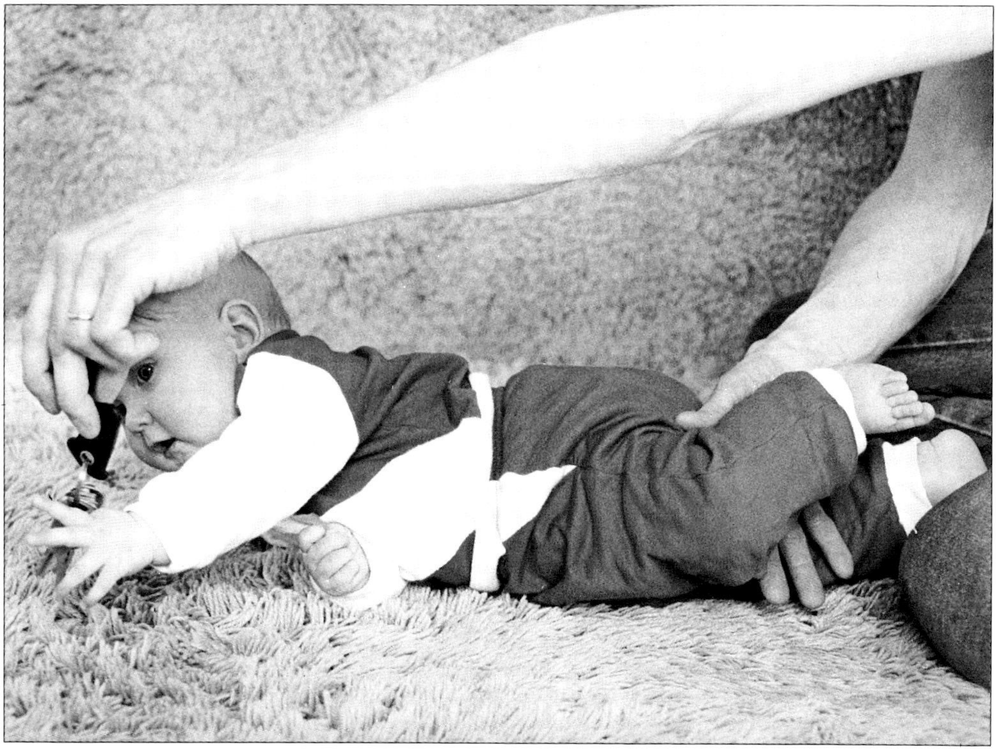

Once your baby discovers her feet, help her gain strength and control of her legs by dangling toys where she can reach them with her toes.

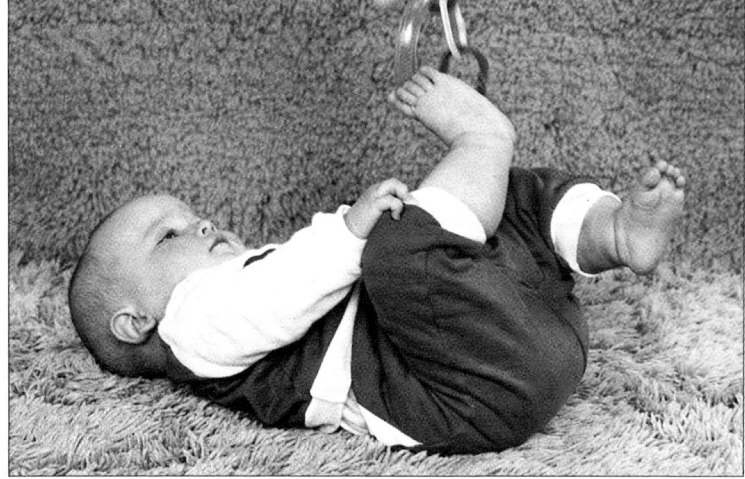

hand behind her left knee, bending it up and pressing the back of your outstretched fingers onto her right thigh to keep it flat. Roll her left hip forward and over toward the right side, waiting for her to follow with her upper trunk and shoulders. When you reverse the movement, tuck her right arm under her chest so that her left shoulder naturally falls backward. Be careful that you are ready to support her head if she needs it, as the movement in this direction is often rather speedy. Don't forget to roll her in the other direction too. This movement will quickly become natural, and you will be able to decrease your assistance as she learns to rotate her body by herself, leading either with an arm or a leg.

Encouraging foot play

At about five months or perhaps a little later, babies have usually begun to learn about their feet by feeling and holding them with their hands, and using them to hit at toys the way they have already learned to do with their hands. This is an important stage of their development as it teaches them body awareness and how to begin controlling their legs.

You can encourage this skill through play. Try holding your baby's hands while suspending a mobile or "cradle gym" above her hips, so that she can easily see it. You may need to arouse her interest by touching her foot against it and making it move or rattle. Now wait and see if she takes her own feet back up to it to play with it herself. She will probably enjoy this activity best if she is lying without wearing a diaper.

Back and arm strengtheners

By about five months babies have enough strength in their backs and arms to take weight on their hands when they lie on their stomachs – their arms lifting their chests off the floor.

You can exercise and further strengthen these important muscles by encouraging your baby first to look at a toy dangled in front of her face and then above her head, and finally to reach for one, all while she is lying on her stomach. To start with she will

The mirror game helps to strengthen your baby's back and neck muscles while amusing her with one of the most fascinating people in her life – herself! Make sure the chest support is as little as necessary, to allow her back muscles to work hard (see page 118).

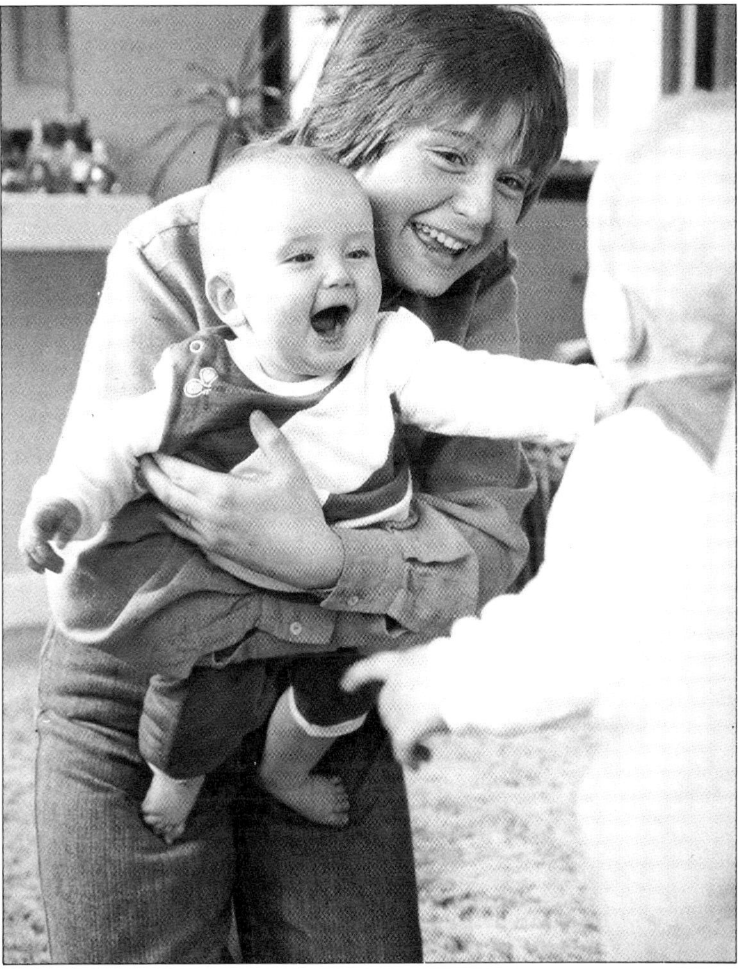

Encourage your baby to push up with straight arms by attracting her attention above her head.

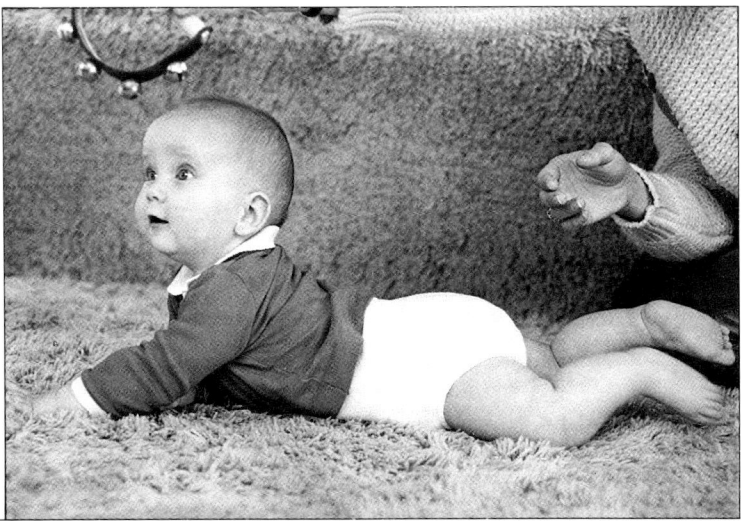

probably only be able to take weight on one straight arm for a brief moment, and reach for a toy on or only just above the ground. As her strength and coordination improve you will be able to hold the toy further up in the air so that she has to reach for it – but never allow her to become frustrated and upset by this game. It should be fun for you both.

Neck and back strengthener

You can further strengthen your baby's neck and back muscles by playing with her in front of a mirror (see page 117). Kneel down holding your baby with her back to you, facing a large mirror. By about five months she will probably like to smile at her own reflection, so give her time to see herself in the mirror before you start. With her feet on your thighs (she will probably enjoy standing on you at this stage), hold one hand in front of her knees and the other supporting her chest, and slowly lower her toward the mirror. Allow her head and back to work as you lower her, giving her minimal support under her chest. She may begin to talk to herself in the mirror. Hold her there as long as she is happy and you are comfortable.

Encouraging your baby to sit

With the increased strength of her back muscles and her strong neck muscles, your baby is now almost ready to sit alone.

When she has begun to learn how to balance, you can try sitting her on the floor between your legs. If she relies on her arms

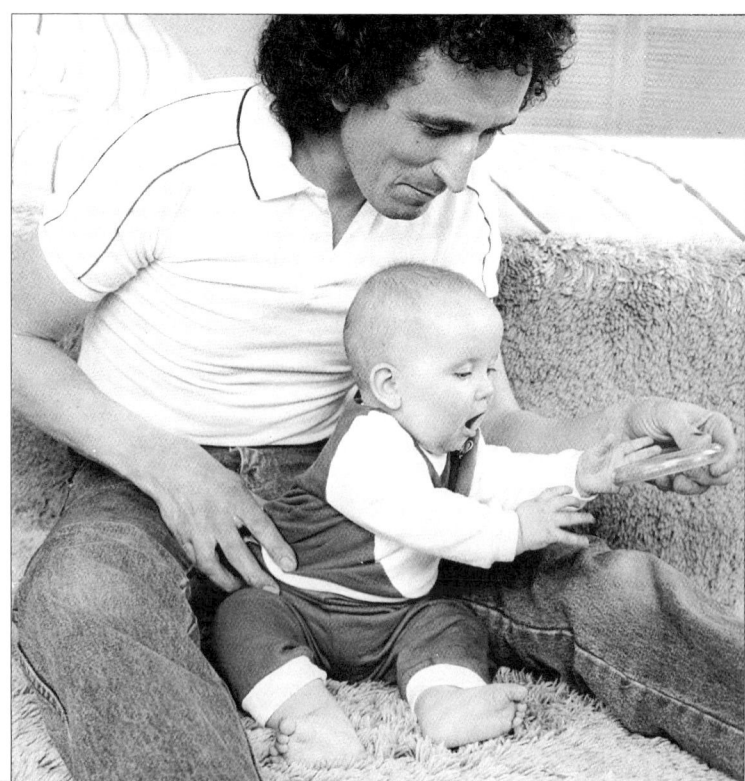

When your baby is almost sitting, play with her on the floor sometimes, so that your legs act as cushions. Once she is able to balance without propping on her arms you can encourage her to reach to either side for a toy.

to prop her up in front, try offering her a toy so that she will reach out with one arm. Gradually she will learn to extend her spine even further and sit up without the help of her arms.

Sitting but not yet safe

By about five to six months your baby will possibly be able to sit up without leaning on her arms, but she will probably not yet have learned the final balance and protective reactions that make sitting alone a stable and safe position. A large cardboard box is the ideal place to put her at this stage; sit her in one corner where the soft sides prevent her falling, and surround her with her favorite toys so she feels safe and secure.

Sitting balance

Once your baby can sit on your knees without support, you can develop her sitting balance further while playing a game. Perhaps to the words of nursery rhymes, like *Ride a Cock Horse* or *Twinkle, Twinkle, Little Star*, you can lift one leg and then the other, starting with small, regular movements, and progressing to larger, less predictable movements, always having your hands free and ready to catch her if she is tipped off balance.

The "parachute reaction"

From about six months, babies learn to "save" themselves when pushed forward while sitting or when lowered head first toward the ground: they react by straightening their arms and putting out their hands to protect their heads. This vital activity is called the "parachute reaction" and can be learned and reinforced in play. If you hold your baby at her trunk and lower her, at first very gently, toward a soft surface such as a bed, she will soon

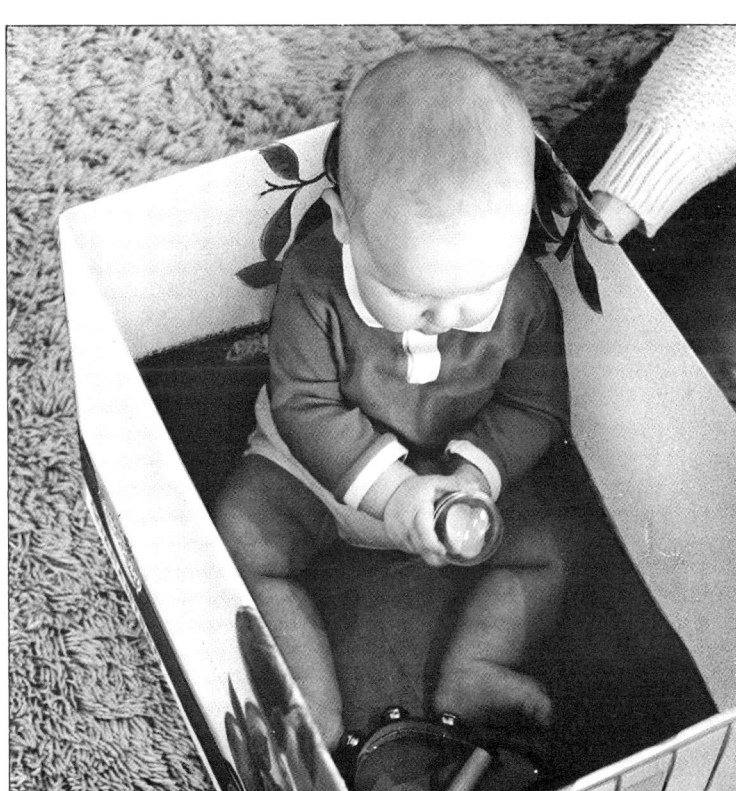

For safety without too much support, let your baby sit and play in a sturdy cardboard box, surrounded by toys.

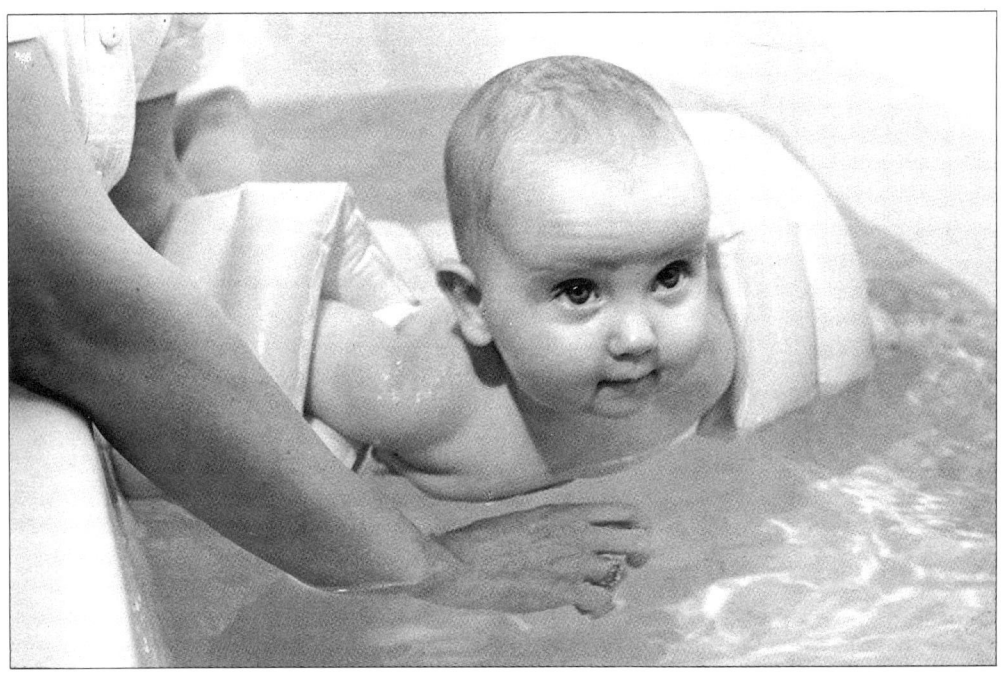

learn to put her arms out, meanwhile straightening her back and lifting her head. This reaction will be particularly important for her early days of walking when she will fall frequently.

Bathtime swimming

Once your baby begins to enjoy her bath, you may like to allow her an occasional "swimming lesson." Run a deep bath and, if you prefer, put inflated arm bands on her upper arms before lowering her into it. Let her kick and splash a little, enjoying the water lapping around her face. Make sure you don't leave her for a second, for obviously she has no sense of self-preservation. It is, and should be, a great game to her, and while she is enjoying herself, she is developing her neck and back muscles but, above all, gaining confidence in the water.

Taking your baby to the swimming pool (see page 122)

After these first "swimming lessons" in the bathtub, you can try taking her to a real swimming pool. Once she has completed her first set of immunizations she will be able to go in the water, provided she is well and the water and air around it warm.

The best way to start is to take your baby into the shallowest part of the pool and just hold her securely, letting her feel the water and absorb her surroundings. Once she is confident, you gently lower her into the pool on her back, supporting her with one open palm under her center of gravity (probably about waist level), while keeping your other forearm and hand under (but not supporting) her neck and head, in case she tips back. Now let her feel the water lapping around her face and body and enjoy the random movements of her limbs.

Above: Bathtime can be the start of swimming lessons. With one hand supporting her waist, let her kick, splash, and blow bubbles. Your free hand is ready to protect her face from accidental immersion.

Once she has good head control, at about five or six months, you can start turning her onto her stomach and supporting her under the chest. She will kick and splash — but watch that she doesn't inhale large amounts of water.

Play and toys

At about three months babies discover their own hands; a few weeks later they learn how to bring them together, to feel objects with them, and to play with rattles that are placed in their hands. By five months they have learned the vital combination of reaching for and getting the thing they see and want, and they then manipulate it, chew it, bang it, and transfer it from hand to hand. By about six months they are sometimes beginning to reach with one hand, and to examine objects very closely.

The toys they need at this stage are few and simple. The first rattle should be one that is bright and attractive, light, well-balanced, and easy to hold in a small fist. It should be safe and pleasurable for biting and mouthing, and make a pleasant noise when moved or shaken. The dumb-bell rattle is an ideal choice, as are teething rings. "Cradle gyms" suspended across the crib or carriage, and activity boards attached to the rails of the crib are worth investing in to amuse your baby. Small soft toys can be fun too. At this age babies like to bring objects up close to their faces, and small soft toys are ideal because they are safe and easy for babies to manipulate. Babies are wonderfully responsive playmates at this stage, but although you will be finding every new development fascinating, you will probably also be pleased to see how much better they are able to occupy themselves for a few minutes with their favorite toys, or just a wooden spoon or some paper to crumple.

Bouncers
and baby walkers

Babies need to learn to roll, rotate their bodies, and move one part or side separately from another as well as simply straightening and pushing with their legs.

Bouncers suspended from door frames can cause babies to develop abnormally persistent stiffness of their legs if they are placed in them for long periods. At the most, fifteen to twenty minutes in a bouncer at any one time is probably all right, provided the baby has plenty of other opportunities to move freely in other positions.

Baby walkers are no longer recommended because they can be dangerous if not closely watched, allowing babies to walk too close to fires and stairs. They can also tip suddenly if they are moving swiftly and meet an obstruction, and might delay natural pre-walking development if overused.

Cribs for the older baby

By now your baby will probably be rapidly outgrowing her first bassinet and you will be ready to move her into a full-size crib. Modern travel cribs may be worth consideration as they are safe, sturdy, and collapsible. However, their mattresses are often very low, so if you have a back problem, the conventional drop-side crib will make lifting your baby out much easier and more comfortable. When choosing a drop-side crib, make sure the movable side has a childproof mechanism for releasing it, and that the bars are no more than $2\frac{1}{2}$ in (6 cm) apart.

Transporting the older baby

As your baby approaches six months, you will find she appreciates outings more, and your own movements will be far less restricted or complicated.

Strollers

The collapsible stroller is now an almost vital addition to your baby equipment – it is so much lighter and more compact than a carriage. Initially you may feel happier if she faces you; as your baby grows you should gradually raise the angle of the seat so that she can look around. She will probably not be able to cope with a stroller in the erect position until she is five to seven months, as she will not have developed the balance reactions in her trunk to keep her upright until then.

Safety car seats

Babies usually have full head control between five and a half and six and a half months; if their bodies are moved they can keep their heads in line and hold them steady. Once the rearward-facing car seat is outgrown, which will depend on your baby's weight, it is safe to put her in a forward-facing seat in the back of the car. This can be secured with a seat belt or attached permanently.

When you are making your choice, make sure that it conforms to U.S. federal safety guidelines, and that it has a buckle that is easy for an adult to master in an emergency, yet not so easy that an inquisitive one-year-old can release it herself. The most effective restraint is a five-point harness that consists of two shoulder straps, a lap belt, and a crotch strap. Do not use a car seat made before the safety guidelines went into effect in 1982.

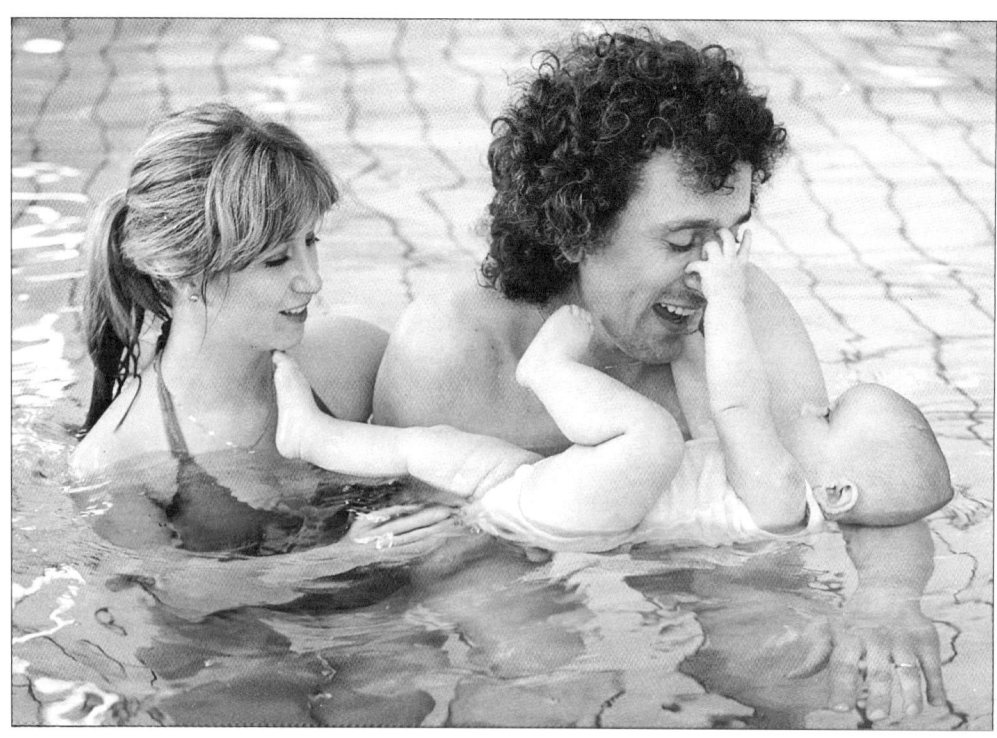

RESUMING NORMAL EXERCISE

If you have been following this exercise program conscientiously, by now not only will your body have recovered fully from the birth of your baby, but you may in fact be fitter than you were before pregnancy. Now you may want to think about maintaining that fitness through sports or other activities.

Making the right choice

Depending on how fit you were before your baby was born, and how regularly you have done your postnatal exercises, you may be able to introduce other sporting activities well before the end of six months. Certainly swimming, walking distances, gentle yoga, and cycling can be started by most women much earlier than activities such as jogging, or aerobics, fitness, and dance classes. Games like tennis and racquetball, and especially squash, require absolute fitness before you start – they are not safe ways of attaining physical fitness. All exercise should be enjoyable and invigorating and should never be taken to the extremes of exhaustion or pain.

Basic advice

1 Don't exercise following a large meal or after drinking alot of fluid.

2 Always warm up and cool down gradually before and after vigorous exercise; in cold weather muscles tend to contract and are more easily damaged, therefore, make sure you are warmly dressed, especially for outside exercise.

3 Make sure that you have the right equipment for your sport – well-padded training shoes for running and loose, comfortable, absorbent clothing.

4 If you're taking up a new sport, such as running or aerobic classes, obtain really sound professional advice as to technique and local facilities. Beware of the unqualified teacher taking classes that are too large to be able to offer individual advice.

5 Don't push yourself beyond your own exercise tolerance; muscle "burning," overstretching, and joint pain can be damaging and may mean you have to rest during a period of recovery.

Swimming

Swimming is an ideal way of getting fit safely. You can start as soon as you have stopped bleeding, though some women prefer to wait until after their postnatal checkup at six weeks. The water can provide both assistance (buoyancy removes the weight of gravity on the body) and resistance, so you can strengthen your muscles and mobilize your joints without the jarring stresses of land sports. If you are still overweight, you are in fact more buoyant, and certain exercises can be easier for you (see page 109).

Once your baby is three to six months old, the whole family can swim together. Hold your baby with one hand under her waist, your other arm submerged and ready to support her head, and she will feel confident in the water.

Simply swimming lengths of a pool is excellent exercise – the heart and lungs are working hard to take oxygenated blood to the muscles. The breast stroke is the most leisurely stroke, but it may aggravate backache; unless you keep your head well down in the water you may overarch your spine. The crawl and backstroke use more energy, and the butterfly is only for the fit person. A relaxed way of swimming is on your back, using breast stroke movements of your legs and supporting arm movements.

Specific exercises to be avoided at all times

1 Lying on your back and lifting both straight legs together.
2 Sit-ups from lying flat with legs straight. (Both numbers 1 and 2 involve risk of damage to your back and your abdominal muscles.)
3 Forced toe-touching whether standing or sitting with legs straight. This can overstretch the spine and hamstring muscles if done in a bouncy, uncontrolled way.
4 "Bicycling" by balancing on your neck and shoulders, or rolling your legs back over your head so your toes touch the ground, can strain and damage the neck and upper back unless your body is well prepared.
5 "Bouncing squats" or "squat thrusts" can damage the knee ligaments and cartilages. It is important to straighten your legs fully between squats.
6 Forcing your thighs apart by sudden pressure with your arms or hands overstretches your tendons and ligaments causing pain, and achieves nothing in terms of fitness. However, if you enjoy the sensation of a good stretch, make sure you allow your soft tissues to lengthen gradually.

Common long-term problems

Even after several months have passed, some women are still bothered by stress incontinence, backache, or painful intercourse. None of these problems should be tolerated because "they are a normal aftereffect of childbirth." They are not and it is well worth consulting a specialist.

Looking forward

We are all different and women's bodies recover from the impact of pregnancy and childbirth at different rates. Exercising regularly in the first six months will help your body regain its pre-pregnancy strength, shape, and firmness, and reequip you for the fun and pleasure of a full and active life, and any sport or activity you previously enjoyed. The rewards of exercising in the early postnatal months are improved posture, stronger, firmer muscles, and a thorough awareness of your pelvic floor. These benefits should be with you for life.

FURTHER READING

Breastfeeding

Dana, N. and Price, Anne, *Successful Breastfeeding: A Complete Step-by-Step Guide to Nursing Your Baby*. Deephaven, Minnesota: Meadowbrook Press, 1985.

Riorday, Janice, *A Practical Guide to Breastfeeding*. Boston, Massachusetts: Jones and Bartlett, 1991.

Sears, W. and Sears, M., *Keys to Breastfeeding*. Hauppauge, New York: Barron's, 1991.

Childcare

Leach, Penelope, *The First Six Months: Getting Together with Your Baby*. New York, New York: Alfred A. Knopf, Inc., 1987.

Sears, W., *Keys to Calming the Fussy Baby*. Hauppauge, New York: Barron's, 1991.

——, *Keys to Preparing and Caring for Your Newborn*. Hauppauge, New York: Barron's, 1991.

——, *Your Baby: The First Twelve Months*. Hauppauge, New York: Barron's, 1989.

Zuckerman, Pamela, *Your Baby: Basic Care and First Aid*. Hauppauge, New York: Barron's, 1987.

Exercise

Noble, E., *Essential Exercises for the Childbearing Year: A Guide to Health and Comfort Before and After Your Baby is Born*. Boston, Massachusetts: Houghton Mifflin, 1988.

Reginer, Susan, *Exercises for Baby and Me*. New York, New York: Simon & Schuster, 1990.

Postnatal Depression

Dalton, Katherine, *Depression after Childbirth: How to Recognize and Treat Postnatal Depression*. New York, New York: Oxford University Press, 1989.

Sapstead, Anne-Marie, *Banish the Post-Baby Blues: All the Advice, Support and Encouragement You Need to Cope*. San Francisco, California: Thorsons Guides, 1990.

USEFUL ADDRESSES

American College of Obstetricians and Gynecologists
409 12th Street SW
Washington, DC 20024

American Foundation for Maternal and Child Health
439 E. 51st Street, 4th Floor
New York, NY 10022

Healthy Mothers, Healthy Babies
409 12th Street SW, Room 309
Washington, DC 20024

International Childbirth Education Association
PO Box 20048
Minneapolis, MN 55420

La Leche League International
PO Box 1209
Franklin Park, IL 60131-8209

National Women's Health Network
1325 G Street NW
Washington, DC 20005

National Maternal and Child Health Clearinghouse
38th and R Streets NW
Washington, DC 20057

INDEX

ACKNOWLEDGMENTS

Margie Polden has worked as an obstetric physiotherapist for nearly forty years. At the Hammersmith Hospital in London, she organizes the all-around physiotherapy care of women during the childbearing year and after. She is a National Childbirth Trust teacher and has four grown children.

Barbara Whiteford is a physiotherapist with specialist training in obstetrics and pediatrics. She has been working in London for twenty-one years, at present teaching pre- and postnatal classes, and assessing and teaching infants with problems in a large West London practice. She has two children.

Author's acknowledgments
The authors would like to thank: Professor Murdoch Elder and the midwives at the Hammersmith Hospital, London, for their advice and for allowing us to use the hospital facilities; Sir George Pinker; Georgina Harris, Niki Medlikova, Erica Hunningher, Caroline Hillier, and Sandra Lousada for their guidance, support, and creativity; and especially our husbands, Iain and Martin.

Medical consultants
David Harvey, M.D., F.R.C.P., Senior Lecturer and Consultant Pediatrician, Queen Charlotte and Chelsea Hospital, London, England.
Concepcion Sia, M.D., Associate Chief, Division of Perinatal Medicine, North Shore University Hospital, Manhasset, New York.

Revisions editor Georgina Harris
Revisions art editor Niki Medlikova
Editor, first revised edition Barbara Vesey

Editor Nicky Adamson
Art editor Caroline Hillier
Designer Anne Fisher
Series editor Pippa Rubinstein
Art director Debbie MacKinnon

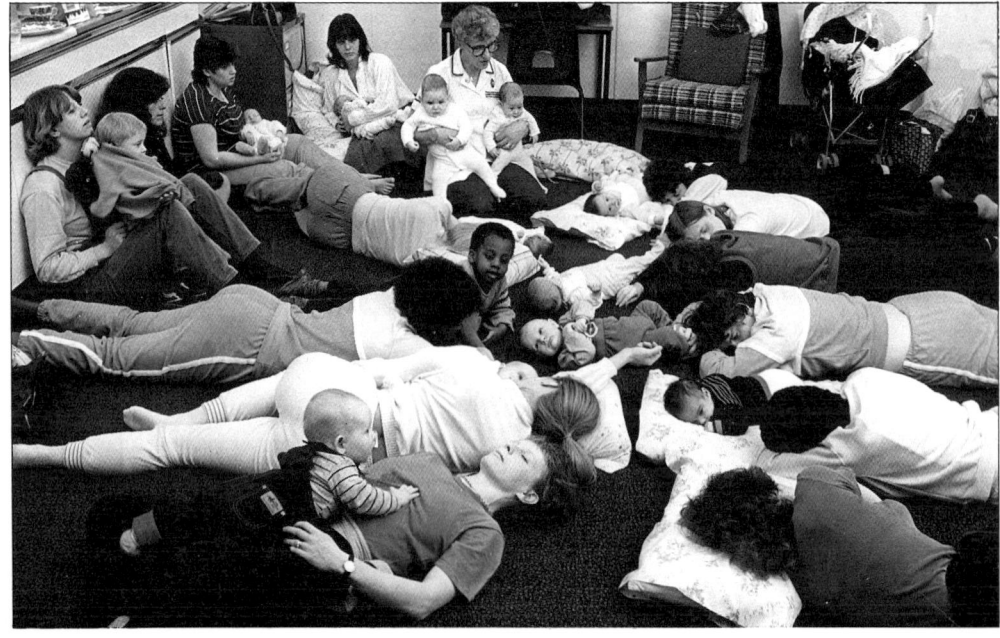